Economic Evaluation in Clinical Trials

Handbooks in Health Economic Evaluation Series

Series editors: Alastair Gray and Andrew Briggs

Existing volumes in the series:

Decision Modelling for Health Economic Evaluation
Andrew Briggs, Mark Sculpher and Karl Claxton

Forthcoming volumes in the series:

Applied Methods of Cost-Effectiveness Analysis
Alastair Gray, James Wolstenholm, Sarah Wordsworth and Philip Clarke

Applied Methods of Cost-Benefit Analysis
Emma McIntosh, Jordan Louviere, Emma Frew and Philip Clarke

Economic Evaluation in Clinical Trials

Dr. Henry A. Glick

Associate Professor of Medicine, Division of General Internal Medicine, School of Medicine; Associate Professor of Health Care Systems, Wharton School; Senior Fellow, Leonard Davis Institute of Health Economics; Associate Scholar, Center for Clinical Epidemiology and Biostatistics, University of Pennsylvania, USA

Dr. Jalpa A. Doshi

Research Assistant Professor of Medicine, Division of General Internal Medicine, School of Medicine; Senior Fellow, Leonard Davis Institute of Health Economics; Associate Scholar, Center for Clinical Epidemiology and Biostatistics, University of Pennsylvania, USA

Dr. Seema S. Sonnad

Associate Professor, Department of Surgery, School of Medicine; Senior Fellow, Leonard Davis Institute of Health Economics; Associate Scholar, Center for Clinical Epidemiology and Biostatistics, University of Pennsylvania, USA

Dr. Daniel Polsky

Associate Professor of Medicine, Division of General Internal Medicine, School of Medicine; Associate Professor of Health Care Systems, The Wharton School; Senior Fellow, Leonard Davis Institute of Health Economics; Associate Scholar, Center for Clinical Epidemiology and Biostatistics, University of Pennsylvania, USA

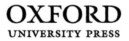

OXFORD
UNIVERSITY PRESS

OXFORD
UNIVERSITY PRESS

Great Clarendon Street. Oxford 0X2 6DP

Oxford University Press is a department of the University of Oxford.
It furthers the University's objective of excellence in research, scholarship,
and education by publishing worldwide in

Oxford New York

Auckland Cape Town Dar es Salaam Hong Kong Karachi
Kuala Lumpur Madrid Melbourne Mexico City Nairobi
New Delhi Shanghai Taipei Toronto

With offices in

Argentina Austria Brazil Chile Czech Republic France Greece
Guatemala Hungary Italy Japan Poland Portugal Singapore
South Korea Switzerland Thailand Turkey Ukraine Vietnam

Oxford is a registered trademark of Oxford University Press
in the UK and in certain other countries

Published in the United States
by Oxford University Press Inc., New York

A catalogue record for this title is available from the British Library

Library of Congress Cataloging in Publication Data

Economic evaluation in clinical trials/Henry A. Glick ... [et al.].
p.; cm. -- (Handbooks in health economic evaluation)
ISBN-13: 978-0-19-852997-2 (pbk.)
ISBN-10: 0-19-852997-x(pbk.)
1. Clinical trials-- Economic aspects. 2. Outcome assessment (Medical care) I. Glick, Henry.
II. Series.
[DNLM: 1. Clincal Trials--economics. 2. Cost-Benefit Analysis--methods. 3. Outcome
Assessment (Health Care)--economics. QV 771 E19 2007]
R853.C55E36 2007
615.5072'4--dc22

2006035981

Typeset by Cepha Imaging Pvt Ltd., Bangalore, India
Printed in Great Britain
on acid-free paper by Biddles Ltd., King's Lynn, Norfolk

ISBN 978–0–19852997–2 (Pbk.)

10 9 8 7 6 5 4 3 2 1

Series preface

Economic evaluation in health care is a thriving international activity that is increasingly used to allocate scarce health resources, and within which applied and methodological research, teaching, and publication are flourishing. Several widely respected texts are already well established in the market, so what is the rationale for not just one more book, but for a series? We believe that the books in the series *Handbooks in Health Economic Evaluation* share a strong distinguishing feature, which is to cover as much as possible of this broad field with a much stronger practical flavour than existing texts, using plenty of illustrative material and worked examples. We hope that readers will use this series not only for authoritative views on the current practice of economic evaluation and likely future developments, but for practical and detailed guidance on how to undertake an analysis. The books in the series are textbooks, but first and foremost they are handbooks.

Our conviction that there is a place for the series has been nurtured by the continuing success of two short courses we helped develop — Advanced Methods of Cost-Effectiveness Analysis, and Advanced Modelling Methods for Economic Evaluation. Advanced Methods was developed in Oxford in 1999 and has run several times a year ever since, in Oxford, Canberra, and Hong Kong. Advanced Modelling was developed in York and Oxford in 2002 and has also run several times a year ever since, in Oxford, York, Glasgow, and Toronto. Both courses were explicitly designed to provide computer-based teaching that would take participants through the theory but also the methods and practical steps required to undertake a robust economic evaluation or construct a decision-analytic model to current standards. The proof-of-concept was the strong international demand for the courses – from academic researchers, government agencies and the pharmaceutical industry – and the very positive feedback on their practical orientation.

So the original concept of the Handbooks series, as well as many of the specific ideas and illustrative material, can be traced to these courses. The Advanced Modelling course is in the phenotype of the first book in the series, *Decision Modelling for Health Economic Evaluation*, which focuses on the role and methods of decision analysis in economic evaluation. The Advanced Methods course has been an equally important influence on *Applied Methods of Cost-Effectiveness*, the third book in the series which sets out the key elements of analyzing costs and outcomes, calculating cost-effectiveness and reporting results. The concept was then extended to cover several other important topic areas. First, the design, conduct, and analysis of economic evaluations along-side clinical trials have become a specialized area of activity with distinctive methodological and practical issues, and its own debates and controversies. It seemed worthy of a dedicated volume, hence the second book in the series, *Economic Evaluation in Clinical Trials*. Next, while the use of cost–benefit analysis in health care has spawned a substantial literature, this is mostly theoretical, polemical, or focused on specific issues such as willingness to pay. We believe the fourth book in the series, *Applied Methods of Cost-Benefit Analysis in Health Care*, fills an important gap in the literature by providing a comprehensive guide to the theory but also the practical conduct of cost–benefit analysis, again with copious illustrative material and worked out examples.

Each book in the series is an integrated text prepared by several contributing authors, widely drawn from academic centres in the UK, the United States, Australia, and elsewhere. Part of our role as editors has been to foster a consistent style, but not to try to impose any particular line: that would have been unwelcome and also unwise amidst the diversity of an evolving field. News and information about the series, as well as supplementary material for each book, can be found at the series website: http://www.herc.ox.ac.uk/books

Alastair Gray   Andrew Briggs
Oxford   Glasgow

July 2006

Web resources

In addition to worked examples in the text, readers of this book can download datasets and programs for Stata for Windows (Stata Corporation, College Station, Texas, U.S) that provide examples of the analysis of cost and QALYs, estimation of sampling uncertainty for the comparison of cost and effect, and calculation of sample size and power for cost-effectiveness analysis in clinical trials.

Materials for the book are maintained at the following web address: www.herc.ox.ac.uk/books/trials.shtml

More information is available at the website. We anticipate that the web-based material will be expanded and updated over time.

Acknowledgment

I first became involved in economic assessment in clinical trials in 1985 when John M. Eisenberg (1946–2002) hired me to manage an economic evaluation for a Veterans Administration (VA) cooperative trial of total parenteral nutrition. I began thinking about the ideas in this book the next year when two events occurred. First, John and I began co-teaching a graduate course in the School of Medicine that eventually was named Medical Decision Making and Clinical Economics. Since 1990, I have co-taught this course with Sankey Williams. Second, Mark Pauly and I began co-teaching Cost-Benefit and Cost-Effectiveness Analysis, a graduate course in the Wharton School. Except for a sabbatical here and there, Mark and I have continued to co-teach it, now with Dan Polsky. John, Mark, Sankey, and Dan have all challenged me and helped me grow both as a researcher and as a person.

I can trace some of the ideas in this book to early lecture notes from these classes. The hundreds of students who have listened to me, questioned me, and made me rethink ways to explain many of the ideas that we present here have all made this a better book than it otherwise would have been.

Other ideas, particularly those in Chapters 5, 8, and 9, were developed as part of research that was supported by the National Institute on Alcohol Abuse and Alcoholism (NIAAA) grant 1 R01 AA12664-01A2 and the National Institute of Drug Abuse (NIDA) grant R01 DA017221-01A1.

Early in my career, Eugene Smith, Joe Heyse, John Cook, Dick Willke, and Martin Backhouse all provided me with funding and opportunities to work on trials. So too did the International Clinical Epidemiology Network (INCLEN). More recently, Mark Bauer gave me the opportunity to lead the economic evaluation of another large VA cooperative trial as have investigators in the NIDDK-funded Look AHEAD and HEALTHY trials. Kevin Schulman was my earliest collaborator, and I think of him as one still. Dan was and is my second collaborator and Jalpa Doshi is the third. Bruce Kinosian and I have worked together since shortly after I began working in the Department of Medicine; Andy Briggs has always had more confidence in me than I deserve. They have all helped me gain whatever success I have had in my career.

My Dad (and my Mom who died in 1984) always had faith in me. I hope they are (would have been) proud. Even though I do not see him, Avivar, my son, brings a smile to my face every day. Finally, there is Seema who helps me through each day. Thank you all.

Henry Glick
July 2006

Table of contents

Chapter 1

Introduction

During the past 30 years, health care expenditures have increased dramatically throughout the world. In the U.S., total national expenditures on health care as a percentage of gross domestic product (GDP) have increased from 7.4% (equivalent to $149 per capita) in 1972 to 15% (equivalent to $5635 per capita) in 2003 [1,2]. Dramatic increases have also taken place in many other developed countries. During this same time period, total expenditures as a percentage of GDP have increased in the United Kingdom from 4.6 to 7.7%, in France from 6.2 to 10.1%, in Germany from 7.1 to 11.1%, and in Japan from 4.8 to 7.90% [1,2].

In response to these increases, countries around the world have been investigating methods to control health care cost. Macro level methods have included greater risk-sharing between payers, providers, and patients as well as a greater reliance on market-oriented incentives. Micro level methods have included making decisions about the utilization of particular medical therapies by government regulators, health care providers, members of formulary committees, payers, and patients based on an evaluation of value for the cost of those therapies.

One potential source of information for decisions about value for the cost derives from clinical trials that establish the efficacy and effectiveness of medical therapies. During the past 20 years, there has been a growing trend to exploit this potential source of information by collecting data on medical service use, cost, and effect in clinical trials. Most frequently economic evaluation has been incorporated into the drug development process, for example in phase III and sometimes phase II, during which a drug's safety and efficacy are evaluated prior to regulatory approval, as well as in phase IV, which occurs after the drug is marketed. Economic evaluations are also increasingly being conducted within trials of other medical therapies such as surgical procedures, behavioral interventions, etc. The U.K. Medical Research Council and U.S. National Institute of Health routinely request the inclusion of economic assessments prior to funding large-scale multicenter trials. Many other countries require evidence of economic value as part of their reimbursement decision making, and clinical trials provide one of the earliest opportunities to generate economic data that can be used for this purpose.

Coincident with this increased attention has been a rapid development in the methodologies used to evaluate the value for the cost of new therapies. More than 20 years ago, most economic evaluations derived from clinical trials were not based on direct observation of the impact of a therapy on cost and effect. Rather, they were based on decision analyses that were developed primarily from epidemiologic data, and borrowed only a few key findings, such as the odds ratio for effectiveness, from the trial. Reported results included point estimates of incremental cost and effect and a point estimate for the cost-effectiveness ratio. Uncertainty was expressed solely by the use of sensitivity analysis.

By the mid-1990s, a growing number of trial-based economic evaluations were based on direct observation of the impact of a therapy on cost and effect. In their 1998 review, Barber and Thompson reported that they identified 45 cost-effectiveness analyses published in 1995 that were based on the analysis of patient-level data that were collected as part of a randomized clinical trial [3]. In these studies, short-term economic impacts of the therapy were directly observed; longer term impacts could potentially be projected by the use of a range of extrapolation methods including decision analytic models.

As with the earlier economic studies, these studies continued to report point estimates of incremental cost and effect, but they also had the opportunity to report confidence intervals for these differences, based on univariate tests of means or multivariable ordinary least squares regression. Most, if not all, of the assessments of value for the cost would have continued to be based on point estimates and sensitivity analysis, in part because the first major article that reported on methods for addressing sampling uncertainty related to cost-effectiveness ratios was published in 1994 [4]. Finally, little to no consideration would have been given to the transferability of the economic results of the trials.

In the past decade, the field has continued to mature. Doshi et al. [5] have reported that in 2003, the number of published economic evaluations that were based on the analysis of patient-level data on cost and effect collected as part of a randomized clinical trial had increased to 115. Sculpher et al. [6] have found that "Since 1994, approximately 30% of published economic evaluations on the NHS Economic Evaluation Database have been based on data from a single RCT" (p. 677). Some studies are now reporting point estimates and confidence intervals for incremental cost, incremental effect, and for the evaluation of value for the cost, for example by reporting the confidence interval for the cost-effectiveness ratio. By this time, the impact of sensitivity analysis on the comparison of cost and effect could be judged by how it affected both the point estimate of the cost-effectiveness ratio or net monetary benefit as well as its effects on the resulting confidence intervals.

The steps involved in conducting an economic evaluation that is incorporated within a randomized trial include: (1) quantification of the cost and effect of care; (2) assessment of whether and by how much average cost and effect differ among the treatment groups; (3) comparison of the magnitudes of differences in cost and effect and evaluation of the "value for the cost" of the therapies, for example by reporting incremental cost-effectiveness ratios; and (4) identifying the populations to whom the results apply. We follow this same structure in the remainder of this volume.

In Chapter 2, we discuss issues related to the design of economic evaluations in trials. We address six study design issues, which include: (1) What preplanning should be done in preparation for the trial? (2) What medical service use should we measure? (3) In what form should the data be collected? (4) Which price weight estimates should be used for the study? (5) How naturalistic should the study design be? and (6) What should we do if the full benefit and cost of therapy are not expected to be observed during the period of observation in the trial? Making sound design decisions about the length of economic follow-up, sample size, minimization of lost-to-follow-up of economic data, collection of adequate amounts of data on medical service use, and the like are essential for trials to provide useful information at their conclusion.

Once data on medical service use are collected, they commonly are translated into measures of cost by multiplying service use times price weights. In Chapter 3, we discuss issues related to the selection of an appropriate set of these weights. Studies commonly use either national or center-specific price weights. Center-specific weights are more likely to provide an estimate of the cost that was incurred in the trial. National price weights are generally considered to be more representative than center-specific weights, particularly for questions of national resource allocation. However, national representativeness of the economic results depends on representative patterns of both medical service use and price weights.

Potential measures of economic effect range from intermediate outcomes, such as blood pressure in millimeters of mercury, to final outcomes, such as length of survival. The Panel on Cost Effectiveness in Health and Medicine [7] has recommended the use of quality-adjusted life years (QALYs) as the principal measure of effect in cost-effectiveness analysis (p. 308). QALYs have the advantages that they combine multiple dimensions of outcome, i.e., survival and quality of life, into a single measure that allows comparisons to be made across therapeutic areas and illnesses and for which we generally understand how much we are willing to pay for a unit of effect. In Chapter 4, we discuss methods for assessing QALYs. In particular we focus on the two most common general approaches to QALY assessment, the use of prescored instruments and direct elicitation methods.

In Chapters 5 and 6, we explore methods for the analysis of cost. In Chapter 5, we discuss strategies for this analysis when we are not concerned about large amounts of censored data; in Chapter 6, we discuss strategies for addressing censored data. The central themes of these chapters are that: (1) the outcome of interest for economic assessment is the difference in arithmetic mean cost (and the difference in arithmetic mean effect), (2) the analytic methods we adopt should estimate and yield inferences about this difference and should not estimate and yield inferences about differences in geometric means or medians, and (3) the evaluation of the difference in arithmetic mean cost is complicated by the fact that the distribution of cost is typically highly skewed with long heavy right tails. As we indicate in Chapter 6, censoring poses additional problems that require diagnosis of the mechanism of censoring and adoption of methods that are appropriate for analysis given the diagnosed mechanism.

Once we have analyzed cost and effect, we compare the two. In Chapter 7, we introduce the two principal methods available for this comparison, the cost-effectiveness ratio and net monetary benefit. In Chapters 8–10, we address two of the potential limitations in the interpretation of the comparison of cost and effect observed in clinical trials. In Chapters 8 and 9, we discuss the concepts underlying the measurement of sampling uncertainty for cost-effectiveness ratios and net monetary benefit (Chapter 8) as well as how to calculate these measures of uncertainty (Chapter 9). Discussion of the latter issue also provides us with the opportunity to address issues of sample size and power for economic evaluations that are incorporated into clinical trials. In Chapter 10, we address the issue of transferability: to whom does the pooled result from the trial apply?

As we indicated above, economic data collected as part of clinical trials are one potential source of information for decisions about value for the cost, but they are not the only potential source of these data. Data from trials and from decision analyses are complementary and have different strengths and weaknesses. We are more certain about what we observed during the trial, but limitations in terms of length of follow-up, treatment comparators, or patient populations studied may mean that the trial does not address all of the considerations that go into treatment adoption decisions. We are less certain about the results from decision analysis, in part, because they either cannot be or have not been formally validated or empirically tested. But these models allow us to address the broader set of considerations that may go into adoption decisions.

There are other volumes in this series that address decision analysis, and they are appropriate for efforts you may make in the development of these models. This volume is intended to provide you with an in-depth understanding of economic assessment conducted by the use of patient-level data collected as part of randomized controlled trials. Our goal is to describe methods that maximize the information we can derive from such patient-level analysis. In doing so, we highlight good practice; we identify commonly misused practices; and in those cases where methods are still rapidly evolving, we summarize the alternative methods.

References

1. Organisation for Economic Cooperation and Development. *OECD Health Data 98.* Paris, France: OECD Electronic Publications, 1998.
2. Organisation for Economic Cooperation and Development. *OECD in Figures, 2005 Edition.* Paris: OECD Publications, 2005.
3. Barber JA, Thompson SG. Analysis and interpretation of cost data in randomised controlled trials: review of published studies. *BMJ.* 1998; 317: 1195–200.
4. O'Brien BJ, Drummond MF, Labelle RJ, Willan A. In search of power and significance: issues in the design and analysis of stochastic cost-effectiveness studies in health care. *Med Care* 1994; 32: 150–63.
5. Doshi JA, Glick HA, Polsky DP. Analyses of cost data in economic evaluations conducted alongside randomized controlled trials. *Value in Health* 2006; 9: 334–40.
6. Sculpher MJ, Claxton K, Drummond M, McCabe C. Wither trial-based economic evaluation for health care decision making? *Health Econ.* 2006; 15: 677–87.
7. Gold MR, Siegel JE, Russell LB, Weinstein MC (eds). *Cost-effectiveness in Health and Medicine.* Oxford: Oxford University Press, 1996.

Chapter 2

Designing economic evaluations in clinical trials

This chapter provides an introduction to issues of design of economic assessments conducted as part of randomized trials. We first describe the gold standard economic evaluation and the tensions that exist in the design of such a study. Second, we discuss six study design issues related to these evaluations. Finally, we address issues such as when it is inappropriate to perform an economic evaluation within a trial and features that contribute to a successful economic evaluation within a trial.

2.1. The gold standard

The gold standard economic evaluation within a clinical trial has a number of defining characteristics. First, it is conducted in naturalistic settings, uses as a comparator a commonly used, cost-effective therapy, and studies the therapy as it would be used in usual care. Second, it is performed with adequate power to assess the homogeneity of economic results in a wide range of clinical settings and among a wide range of clinical indications in which the therapy will be used. Third, it is designed with an adequate length of follow-up to assess the full impact of the therapy. Fourth, it is conducted within a timeframe that allows the resulting information to provide important decisions in the adoption and dissemination of the therapy.

In a gold standard evaluation, we measure all cost of all participants in the trial regardless of why the cost was incurred, starting prior to randomization and continuing for the duration of follow-up of the trial. Cost incurred after randomization constitutes the cost outcome of interest in the trial (at least for the period of observation within the trial; in some cases, we may also want to project cost and effect beyond this period of observation). Cost incurred prior to randomization is a potential predictor of cost after randomization, and thus may explain variability in this cost.

Given that in the gold standard we measure all cost, we measure the cost that is believed to be related to the disease and its treatment as well as the cost that might be expected to be unrelated. We do so because the gold standard evaluation is adequately powered; thus, rather than making judgments about the relationship between therapy and a particular medical service, we empirically determine the incremental cost that is related to the therapy. This measurement of all cost has implications for the debate about whether or not the evaluation should include only that cost that is related to the intervention or whether it should include "unrelated" cost as well [1,2].

Issues related to the type of analysis that will be conducted, for example cost–benefit, cost-effectiveness, or cost-minimization analysis, apply equally to economic evaluations that are incorporated within clinical trials (be they gold standard evaluations or otherwise) as they do to other economic evaluations. So too do issues related to the types of cost that will be included, for example direct medical, direct nonmedical, productivity, and intangible, and the perspective from which the study will be conducted. These issues have been well addressed in the literature [3–5], and we do not discuss them further.

Performing a gold standard evaluation is most feasible when it is easy to identify when services are provided, for example in hospital-based studies or studies conducted within integrated systems of care. Feasibility is also enhanced when medical service use and cost data are already being collected, for example in an administrative database, and when researchers have ready access to these data once they are collected. Traditionally, hospital-based studies have been considered as some of the best candidates for gold standard studies, because of the closed nature of the hospital, and because of the large amounts of record-keeping that are carried out there. However, as episodes of care increasingly continue after discharge from the hospital, and when some types of medical service use are not collected as part of the administrative record, for example physician cost in the U.S., even these studies fail to meet the standard.

At the same time, the requirements of gold standard assessments pose several drawbacks and feasibility issues. First, there may be contradictions between the goal related to conducting the trial in naturalistic settings and the one related to providing information within a timeframe that informs important decisions. The information from trials that are performed early in the life of a therapy, for example during phases II and III of the drug development process, may aid decisions about early adoption and diffusion of the therapy. If the therapy is dramatically effective, these trials may also be one of the last chances we have to randomize patients to receive the therapy, because once information about a therapy's clinical effectiveness is available, patients may not be willing to participate in experiments simply to evaluate its value for the cost. These early trials, however, may not reflect the cost and effect that would be observed in usual practice, in part because, due to regulatory needs, the trials may affect usual practice and in part because clinicians may not yet know how to use the therapy efficiently.

Trials that are performed later, such as post-marketing studies in the drug development process, are more capable of reflecting usual practice, although it is possible that – due to formal protocols – such trials reduce observed variation in practice. However, information from these trials may be too late to inform important early decisions about the adoption and diffusion of the therapy, and as noted above, if the therapy is shown to be clinically effective, patients may be unwilling to enroll in them. To address some, but not all, of these issues, ideally, we would evaluate new therapies throughout the development process, to inform early decisions and to reevaluate economic findings once the therapy is in common use.

A second feasibility issue is that the need for adequate power in gold standard economic evaluations may require a larger number of study participants than the investigators or funders are willing to enroll. Third, such evaluations may require a longer follow-up than that required for clinical endpoints; for example the economic impacts of therapy may not end at 28 days, but regulatory agencies may accept clinical endpoints measured at 28 days as evidence of clinical efficacy. Finally, the additional burden of economic data collection may exacerbate the problem that some investigators already face in collecting the clinical data required by a trial. Reconstructing the equivalent of a patient bill in the case report form is burdensome. Also, investigators may have limited access to information on medical services provided to study participants from providers and in centers that are unaffiliated with the trial.

Because of these limitations, investigators often make trade-offs between the ideal economic assessment and assessments that are most feasible under the presumption that imperfect information is better than none.

2.2. Six study design issues

When designing a study, we need to consider at least six sets of issues. These include: (1) What preplanning should be done in preparation for the trial? (2) What medical service use – also referred to as resource use – should we measure? (3) In what form should the data be collected? (4) Which price weight – also referred to as unit cost – estimates should be used for the study? (5) How naturalistic should the study design be? and (6) What should we do if the full benefit and cost of therapy are not expected to be observed during the period of observation in the trial?

2.2.1. What preplanning should be done in preparation for the trial?

A number of preplanning activities should be performed when designing an economic assessment within a clinical trial. These include, but are not limited to, identifying an appropriate length of follow-up for economic endpoints; estimating arithmetic means, variances, and correlations for cost, health-related quality of life, and preference; identifying the types of medical services used by study participants; pilot testing data collection instruments and procedures; and gauging levels of patient interest in the study.

Identifying an appropriate length of follow-up for economic endpoints

Economic assessments conducted as part of randomized trials are meant to allow decision makers to use the results of the trial to reach conclusions about the economic benefits of the therapy under investigation. One design issue that may limit the interpretability of the economic data collected within the trial is the study's time horizon. Although clinical efficacy may be demonstrated when a difference in clinical endpoints is observed between study arms, from an economic perspective the appropriate time horizon for a trial would include all or a substantial portion of the time when there is medical service use related to the illness under study. The economic time horizon that would best inform decision makers about the value for the cost of a therapy thus need not be the same as the one adopted for answering the clinical question.

A number of approaches are available for identifying an appropriate economic time horizon for a clinical trial. One approach is to identify the economic episode of care. As defined in the literature, an episode of care is the period initiated by patient presentation with a diagnosis of a clinical condition, or in the case of a randomized trial, initiated by randomization, and concluded when the condition is resolved [6–9]. For definition of the clinical episode, resolution may refer to the acute clinical condition; for definition of the economic episode, it may refer to the return of cost or other outcomes such as preference for current health to the level that would have existed had the clinical condition not been present [10].

Mehta *et al.* [11] and Schulman *et al.* [12] have used episode of care methodology to define economic episodes of care for diabetic foot ulcers [11] and migraine headaches [12]. These authors quantified the length of an economic episode by comparing differences in mean daily cost and differences in the proportion of patients with cost before and after an index diagnosis of foot ulcer and migraine headache: the episode was said to last until the initially elevated mean cost per day (proportion of patients with cost) after the diagnosis returned to their level prior to the diagnosis.

Figure 2.1 shows the mean daily cost for 60 days prior to an index diagnosis of migraine (days −60 to −1), the mean cost during the day of the index diagnosis (day 0), as well as mean daily cost for the 60 days after the index

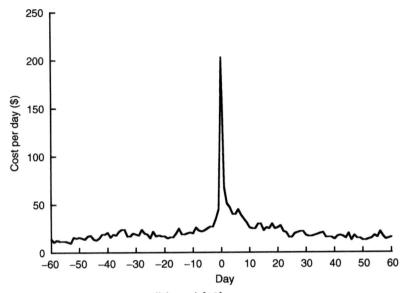

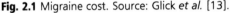

Fig. 2.1 Migraine cost. Source: Glick *et al.* [13].

Source: Reproduced from Glick HA, Polsky D, Schulman K. Trial-based Economic Evaluations: An Overview of Design and Analysis. Chapter 6 Drummond M, McGuire (eds) Economic Evaluation in Health Care. Merging Theory and Practice, Oxford University Press, 2001, 113-40 by permission of Oxford University Press.

diagnosis (days 1 to 60). Analysis of the data suggested that cost from a migraine headache may remain elevated for 3 weeks [12], which is markedly longer than clinical time horizons for migraine therapies, which often can be as short as 30 – 120 min. Given that the economic evaluation is meant to identify both the clinical and economic impacts of therapies, in this case for the treatment of migraine, we would be more likely to capture the latter effects by lengthening the time horizon of the trial and studying the entire period of time when cost is elevated.

Decision analysis represents the second approach that can be adopted for identifying an appropriate economic time horizon for a clinical trial [14]. For example, a decision analytic model that simulates the disease and the effects of therapy might demonstrate that life expectancy among individuals who would have died without the intervention but now live because of it has a substantial impact on the economics of the therapy. In this case, the time horizon of the trial could be adjusted so that we are able to assess these gains in life expectancy, or we could ensure that data are collected that would allow the prediction of life expectancy after the trial.

Estimating arithmetic means, variances, and correlations for cost, health-related quality of life, and preference

Arithmetic means, variances, and correlations for cost, health-related quality of life, and preference provide the information necessary for assessing the sample size required to answer the economic questions posed in the study. Enrollment size for randomized trials often is based on the minimum number of study participants needed to address the clinical questions. However, the number of participants required for the economic assessment may differ from that needed for the clinical evaluation.

Prior to the development of the literature that described confidence intervals for cost-effectiveness ratios [15–19], a common approach to sample size calculation for economic evaluation in trials was to select the larger of the sample sizes needed for estimating pre-specified cost and effect differences. For example, what sample size was required to identify a difference in cost of 1000, and what was required to identify a 10% reduction in mortality?

The development of this literature made it clear, however, that the goal of economic evaluation in trials was to determine whether we can be confident about a therapy's value for the cost. Thus, current sample size methods base their calculations on the number of study participants needed to rule out unacceptably high cost-effectiveness ratios or, alternatively, to rule out that the net monetary benefits of the intervention are less than 0. See Chapter 9 for formulas for sample size and power.

These methods generally require more information than is needed for estimating sample sizes for clinical outcomes or for cost differences alone. Basic data for such calculations include the magnitude of the incremental cost and effect we expect to observe in the trial; the standard deviations for cost and effect in each of the treatment groups; our willingness to pay for health, for example 30,000 or 50,000 per QALY; and the correlation between the difference in cost and effect.

Where do we obtain this information on means, standard deviations, and correlations? If both therapies are already in use, expected differences in outcome and standard deviations can be derived from feasibility studies or from records of patients like those who will be enrolled in the trial. In addition, at least one study has suggested that the correlation between cost and effect observed in these data may be an adequate proxy for the correlation between the difference in cost and effect [15]. For novel therapies, on the other hand, which have yet to be used in large numbers of patients, information about the magnitude of the incremental cost and effect may not be available, and thus may need to be generated by assumption. Data on the standard deviations for those who receive usual care/placebo again may be obtained from feasibility studies or from patient records. We may assume that the standard deviation thus obtained will apply equally to both treatment groups, or we may make alternative assumptions about the relative magnitudes of these deviations. The observed correlation between cost and effect might again be used as a proxy for the correlation between the differences.

In some instances, the economic outcome may have less power than the clinical outcome. In this case, power calculations can be used to assess the magnitude of the cost and effect differences that can be detected. However, due to the fact that economic outcomes are joint outcomes of cost and effect, it is also possible for them to have more power than clinical outcomes [20]. For example, it is possible for the p-value for the difference in both cost and effect to be greater than 0.05, yet for us to confidently conclude that the ratio falls below 30,000 or 50,000 or, alternatively, that net monetary benefit – calculated by use of a willingness to pay of 30,000 or 50,000 – is significantly greater than 0.

The discussion on sample size for addressing economic questions has implications for the selection of endpoints for the economic study. As indicated, determination of sample size requires that we be able to specify what we are willing to pay for a unit of health effect. Debate remains about willingness to pay for a QALY [21–24], the currently recommended outcome for cost-effectiveness analysis [5]. When researchers use disease-specific measures of effect such as cases of disease detected, or in alcohol research, abstinence days, or in many fields, symptom-free days, it is even less clear how much we should be willing to pay for these outcomes. While we can calculate a cost-effectiveness ratio for any outcome we want, to be convincing that a more costly and more effective therapy is of good value, the outcome must be one for which we have recognized benchmarks of cost-effectiveness. These considerations argue against use of too disease-specific an outcome for economic assessment.

As an example, Gupta reported that in comparison with a topical antifungal agent, one triazole antifungal agent cost $5.67 per toenail fungus symptom-free day, while a second triazole compound cost $8.88 per symptom-free day [25]. Without an idea of the value of a toenail fungus symptom-free day, it is not clear whether we should reject both of the triazole antifungal agents, for example if our willingness to pay is less than $5.67; adopt the less expensive and less effective of the two triazole compounds if our willingness to pay ranges between $5.67 and $8.888; or adopt the higher cost, more expensive triazole compound if our willingness to pay is greater than or equal to $8.88.

Identifying the types of medical services used by study participants

A third preplanning activity is to identify the types of medical services that are likely to be used by study participants. We can do so by reviewing medical charts or administrative data sets; having patients keep logs of their medical service use; or asking patients and experts about the kinds of care received by those with the condition under study. This information will help answer questions about the medical service use that should be measured (see discussion in next section), particularly if, because of the burden of economic data collection, only a subset of medical services are to be recorded in case report forms. While analysis of administrative data may provide good estimates of the types of medical services that are used in current practice, we must also be prepared to collect data on additional services to account for the fact that new therapies may change practice, for example by causing adverse outcomes that require different kinds of services than are used by study participants in usual practice.

Pilot testing data collection instruments and procedures

As with any other forms and procedures used in clinical trials, those used to collect economic data should be pilot tested for their efficiency, clarity, and ease of use. Poorly designed forms can lead to low-quality data that will jeopardize our ability to draw useful conclusions from the study.

Gauging levels of patient interest in the study

Substantial amounts of data may be collected from study participants, for example medical service use from providers and in centers that are unaffiliated with the trial, quality of life data, and measures of patient preference, and the amount that is feasible to collect will depend on the level of the participants' interest in the study. This level of interest potentially varies from disease to disease, and gauging it allows investigators to better estimate how much data collection the study participants' will tolerate.

2.2.2. What medical service use should we measure?

In a trial that provides ready access to administrative data, for example from insurers, government agencies, or hospitals, few if any tradeoffs need to be made about the proportion of medical service use – and thus cost – that should be measured in the study. However, if data on this use will be collected prospectively in study case report forms, then the goals are to (1) measure services that make up a large portion of the difference in treatment between study participants randomized to the therapies under evaluation – sometimes referred to as cost "drivers" – and (2) measure services that make up a large portion of the total cost of care. The former services provide an estimate of the new therapy's impact on the cost of care; the latter services provide a measure of overall variability of cost. In addition, failure to measure a large portion of the total cost of care leaves the study open to criticisms that differences in measured services observed between therapies may have been offset among services that were not measured in the study.

The best approach is to measure as many services as possible, because minimizing the services that go unmeasured reduces the likelihood that differences among them will lead to study artifacts. However, there are neither a priori guidelines about how much data are enough, nor data on the incremental value of specific items in the economic case report form. Decisions about those procedures that will be recorded within the case report form and those that will not should take into account the expense of collecting particular data items.

We can obtain information to guide these decisions if, during the preplanning process, we identify the types of medical services that are used by patients who are similar to the patients who will be enrolled in the trial. In general, however, substantially more experience with various medical problems and interventions will be needed before we know which data are essential to document in an economic case report form.

The root of the concern about the amount and type of medical service use that should be collected within a trial is that there may be insufficient resources to identify all medical service use among all participants. In contrast to the general advice above, several alternative strategies have been proposed for rationalizing the amount of data that are collected for the calculation of cost. These include: limiting data collection to those services that health care providers deem are related to the illness or therapy under study; limiting data collection to medical services provided by the study site; and limiting the number of participants for whom economic data are collected. While all the three have the strength of reducing resources required for data collection, most if not all have the cost of potentially undermining what can be learned from the economic evaluation.

Limit data collection to disease-related services

In cases where we do not expect to affect all medical service use, we may be concerned (1) about the cost of collecting "unrelated" service use and (2) that the variability introduced by collecting "unrelated" service use may make it more difficult to detect differences that are expected from "related" service use. One proposed solution to this problem is to limit data collection to disease-related services.

Limiting data collection via this method may succeed in reducing both the cost of the trial and the variability that is introduced into our estimate of cost by collecting all services of certain types, independent of the reason for these services. However, there potentially are several problems with this strategy. For example, there is little if any evidence about the accuracy, reliability, or validity of judgments about what is and what is not disease related. Much of medical practice is multifactorial. In a trial for heart failure, a participant with more severe heart failure may be hospitalized for a comorbid condition, whereas a participant with the same comorbidity, but with milder heart failure may not be hospitalized. Answering counterfactuals such as "would the participant have been hospitalized had his or her heart failure been other than it is?" is the role of randomized trials, and it is unclear that provider judgment is any better at answering questions about the reasons for treatment than they are at answering questions about overall treatment efficacy.

In addition, for participants with complicated conditions, procedures ordered for the diagnosis and treatment of one condition may be complements or substitutes for procedures ordered for other conditions. Thus, even if providers are certain that they are ordering tests or procedures for the illness or therapy under study, it is possible that the same tests or procedures would have been ordered later for different reasons.

While these two limitations argue against collecting only that medical service use which is considered to be disease related, they do not argue against identifying those services that are or are not judged to be disease related. One can then perform a secondary analysis that evaluates cost differences that are stratified by these judgments.

Limit the delivery settings in which medical service use is collected

It is usually less costly to collect information about medical service use when study participants see study personnel in study centers than it is when they see nonstudy providers in centers that are unaffiliated with the trial. Given the relatively higher cost of collecting data in the latter settings compared with the former, some may propose to eliminate collection of data from nonstudy providers and sites. However, ignoring the cost of nonstudy center care may lead to the conclusion that one treatment group has a higher cost than another, when in truth cost among the groups is similar, but incurred in different settings. Thus, if large amounts of care are provided in these settings, or if there are reasons to believe that utilization in these settings will differ among treatment groups, we should consider extending data collection efforts to these settings.

Presuming that the study is designed to collect data on service use from providers and in centers that are unaffiliated with the trial, a strategy should be in place to identify when study participants receive these services. This information may be easy to collect if administrative data such as insurance records are available for the study population or if they receive the preponderance of care from study investigators. In other cases, however, the data will have to come from – sometimes fallible – reporting by study participants or study participants' proxies.

If the data come from study participants or proxies, a decision should be made about how often study participants will be contacted. The more frequently they are interviewed, the less likely the data will be affected by recall bias; however, the cost of data collection is higher and the burden on study participants and proxies is greater. The less frequently they are interviewed, the cost of the data is lower and the burden is lessened. The data, however, are more likely to be affected by recall bias. For example, one study found that 10% of patients failed to report that they had been hospitalized when they were interviewed approximately 5 months after their discharge; another found that 50% failed to report them 10–11 months after their admission [26].

Even if study participants remember that they have seen a physician or have gone to a hospital, they often will not know what services they received. Options for identifying these services include contacting the care providers directly or assuming a standard set of services, such as the marginal cost for a usual visit to a family physician. Standard sets of services might be assigned differentially to account for differences by indication, for example diagnosis-related group; differences in duration, for example brief versus intermediate office visits; or the presence of an intensity marker such as a major diagnostic study.

When collecting data from study participants, another issue is whether to simply rely on their memory or whether to have each study participant use a memory aid, such as a diary [27]. Diary forms can be actual pages in the case report form. More commonly, they are aids that are provided to the participant which are reviewed or abstracted by study personnel so the information can be coded on the case report form. If diaries are used, the investigators should decide how often to contact each study participant with a reminder to use the diary.

Lastly, who will collect these data: the research staff at the study site or a contract research organization? Contract research organizations can often provide interviewers and computerized interview scripts with built-in skip logic and on-line data entry. On the other hand, the study-site research staff sometimes is wary of having outside organizations contacting their patients, particularly if the patients have a stigmatizing disease. However, these same staff may be pleased to avoid having to interview their patients about medical service use on a regular basis.

Limit participants from whom economic data are collected

A third method of reducing data collection cost is to limit the number of participants from whom these data are collected. If, however, there is the same or less power for the economic endpoints than there is for the clinical endpoints, such a strategy will limit the confidence we will have in the study's conclusions.

If there is more power for the economic than the clinical endpoints, we might choose to limit the number of subjects for whom economic data are collected. In this case, the data should come from a random sample of all study participants. Nonrandom sampling, on the other hand, is problematic. For example, in an effort to speed completion of the trial, investigators might enroll participants who agree to participate in the trial but are unwilling to cooperate with the economic assessment. Such an approach can be problematic because self-selection by study participants places the validity of the economic study in jeopardy. The economic assessment could end up comparing an estimate of effects from the entire study population with an estimate of cost derived from a relatively small and nonrandom subset of the population.

Another approach to reducing data collection burden is to limit the economic assessment to the study centers that elect to participate. Unfortunately, this approach can also lead to difficulties. In one study that used voluntary data collection [28], the average length of stay (LOS) among study participants at centers that provided supplementary data was not the same as the average stay from nonresponding centers. This difference made the data analysis substantially more complex in that we could not analyze LOS in the ICU directly, but instead had to impute it based on LOS in the hospital and other explanatory factors.

In summary, the general strategy we recommend is to identify types of medical services that will be documented within the case report form (e.g., hospitalization) and then to collect all of these services independent of their cause. Of note, the fact that we collect this service use without regard to its cause does not mean we do not record information such as primary and secondary diagnoses for inpatient stays that may be used to help cost out these stays (see discussion in Chapter 3). As in the gold standard evaluations, this strategy allows randomization to determine those services that are and are not related to the study therapy. Unless we have a priori hypothesis that differences will be found among low-cost medical services, we recommend that attention be given to high-cost services that are likely to make up a large portion of total cost. For example, for heart failure, we might focus on hospitalization – for severe heart failure we might also focus on outpatient visit cost; for hospitalized infections, we might focus on intensive, intermediate, and routine care unit LOS and major procedures; and for asthma, we might focus on hospitalizations, emergency department visits, and comedications.

During preplanning, we can develop means of reducing data collection cost, without undermining the validity of the results, by identifying those services that are likely to make up a large portion of the difference in cost between the treatment groups. If we determine that the therapy is likely to affect the number of hospitalizations, collect information that will provide a reliable estimate of the cost of these hospitalizations. If it is likely to affect days in the hospital and location in the hospital, collect this information. If the therapy is principally likely to affect outpatient care, collect measures of outpatient care, and the like.

2.2.3. At what level should medical service use be aggregated?

A strategy commonly adopted for calculating cost in trials is to count medical service use that occurs during the trial and to multiply this count by a set of price weight estimates for these services. The level at which medical services are aggregated – for example for inpatient care, should we count hospitalizations? days in the hospital stratified by location in the hospital? should we in addition count individual services provided in the hospital – and the resulting price weight estimates required for the calculation of cost, depend on a number of factors, including whether we expect the intervention to affect the number of hospitalizations that occur, the LOS of a hospitalization when it occurs, or the intensity of medical services utilized during the stay. In making decisions about the level of aggregation at which the data will be collected, the investigator should consider the likely difference more or less aggregated information will have on the study result as well as the cost of collecting more or less aggregated data.

At the most aggregate level, outpatient care can be recorded as the number of visits. Alternatively, diagnostic tests, procedures, and treatments can be recorded as well. For hospital care, the types of services that are counted – and the resulting price weight estimates required for the calculation of cost – often depend on the setting in which the therapies under investigation are expected to be used. For therapies used predominantly in hospital settings, a common approach is to sum the individual costs of a hospital stay, such as those associated with days in the hospital, stratified by intensity of care, laboratory evaluations, procedures, and medications, [28–31].

For therapies used predominantly in outpatient settings, it is more common to collect information about hospital diagnoses and LOS. These hospitalizations can be valued by use of aggregate measures of hospital cost, such as diagnosis-related group (DRG) payments [31–36] or an estimate of the cost per day times the number of days in the hospital [37–39]. When this latter strategy is adopted, different studies may use cost estimates with varying levels of specificity. For example, one of the least specific approaches would be to use a single cost estimate from a single center to value all hospitalizations at all centers, whereas one of the most specific would be to use diagnosis-specific price weight estimates from each center that participated in the study. Most studies adopt a strategy that falls somewhere between these extremes.

2.2.4. **Which price weight estimates should be used for the study?**

Sources of price weights differ by country. For example, in the United States, there are a number of publicly available sources, including hospital charges adjusted using cost-to-charge ratios; data from internal hospital costing systems; DRG payments for hospitalizations [41]; and resource-based relative value units for physician services [41,42].

Readily available data in Europe and in some other parts of the world may include, depending on the country: fee schedules; data from DRG studies; and data from hospital costing systems. In some cases, data have been obtained from a limited number of centers which have cost accounting systems or from administrative databases that recently have been developed in some countries [43].

It may also be possible to develop trial-specific costing exercises, for example analysis of accounting data [44,45], time and motion studies [46], or cost allocation projections for expensive experimental capital equipments [47].

Detailed discussion related to the development of price weights for the evaluation is provided in Chapter 3.

2.2.5. **How naturalistic should the study design be?**

Given that the primary purpose of cost-effectiveness analysis is to inform real-world decision-makers about how to respond to real-world health care needs, the more naturalistic the trial, in terms of participants, analysis based on the intention to treat, and limitation of loss to follow-up, the more likely the data developed within the trial will speak directly to the decision question. Often, however, trials adopt less naturalistic study designs or do not actively seek to limit loss to follow-up. Effects of these decisions are discussed below.

Sample inclusion criteria

First, many phase III efficacy trials and some effectiveness trials employ stringent inclusion and exclusion criteria, and may employ cream skimming – the selection of a subset of the healthiest eligible patients – or reverse cream skimming – the selection of a subset of the sickest eligible patients – in the construction of their study sample. The resulting sample may not represent the more heterogeneous population found in general practice that decision-makers consider when making resource allocation decisions. The efficacy, effectiveness, and efficiency of therapies may be different in the more homogeneous set of participants included in the trial as compared to patients in the general population, and – the arguments of decision analysts to the contrary – it is not clear that valid and reliable data are available to enable translation from what was observed in the homogenous sample to what would have been observed in the heterogeneous one.

Intention-to-treat analysis

Second, given that in real-world settings, economic questions relate to treatment decisions, for example whether to prescribe a therapy, not whether the patient received the therapy prescribed nor whether, once they started the prescribed therapy, they were switched to other therapies, cost and benefit associated with these later decisions should be attributed to the initial treatment decision. Thus, trial-based cost-effectiveness analyses should adopt an intention-to-treat design.

Loss to follow-up

Third, we should design studies in such a way that they minimize the occurrence of missing and censored data. For example, study designs should include plans to aggressively pursue subjects and data throughout the trial. One long-term study of treatment for bipolar disorder was designed from the outset to respond to missed interviews by (1) intensive outreach to reschedule the assessment followed by (2) telephone assessment followed by (3) interview of a proxy who had been identified and consented at the time of randomization [48].

Investigators should also ensure that follow-up continues until the end of the study period. As Polsky *et al* [48] have argued, data collection should not be discontinued simply because a subject reaches a clinical or treatment stage such as failure to respond (as, for example, happens in some antibiotic, cancer chemotherapy, and psychiatric drug trials). This last recommendation may conflict with some commonly used efficacy designs that are event-driven and end follow-up when a participant reaches such a stage. However, given that failure often is associated with a change in the pattern of cost, for example due to the initiation of alternative therapies and the potential elongation of the duration of the episode of care or due to the discontinuation of all treatments, discontinuation of these participants from the economic study is likely to bias the results of an economic evaluation that is conducted as part of the trial.

In general, bias related to follow-up is least likely to occur if all study participants are followed for a fixed time period, for example all study participants are followed for 1 year after randomization or until death, whichever is sooner. Another design which is unbiased – but, as discussed in Chapter 6, requires the use of analytic methods for addressing censored data – is to end follow-up on a given calendar date, for example when the 500th death is observed in the trial. This design, which has been used in a number of long-term cardiovascular trials [49,50], gives rise to what is called "administrative censoring" and the resulting data are usually classified as being "missing completely at random" [51].

Protocol-induced cost and effect

Finally, clinical trial protocols often try to standardize the care of participants in the trial. In doing so, they may require a substantial number of investigations and diagnostic tests that would not be performed under normal clinical practice. They may also prescribe aggressive documentation and treatment of the outcomes observed in the trial.

A common reaction is to exclude the cost of protocol-induced services from the economic evaluation, in part because it is argued that they would not have occurred in usual practice. However, when they have little or no impact on care of participants, exclusion of these services is not particularly important, and when they affect care, it may be difficult if not impossible to exclude the full impact of these services from the analysis.

Take, for example, a protocol-required maneuver that would not commonly be performed in usual practice and which has little or no impact on clinical care. Such care usually represents the simple addition of a constant to our cost estimates. Thus, while its inclusion or exclusion affects the arithmetic mean cost for each treatment group, it will have little effect on the difference between the cost of therapies.

If, on the other hand, this same maneuver would have been performed in some participants, but not in others, the fact that it is mandated for all participants will bias the cost analysis to the null. In this case, we can no longer observe a difference that might have existed between the groups. Unlike the first example, inclusion or exclusion of this cost makes little difference not because it represents a constant, but because neither option can correct the bias that may have been induced by the protocol.

There are at least two more pernicious forms of protocol-induced services whose full impact cannot be corrected by simply excluding the service cost itself. First, suppose a protocol calls for more active monitoring for either outcomes or adverse events than would occur in usual practice, for example, when monitoring for cases of malaria in the evaluation of treated bed nets, for deep vein thrombosis after elective hip replacement, or for nephrotoxicity for certain antibiotics. Such monitoring can lead to the detection of more outcomes than would have been detected in usual care, with the attendant increase in cost associated with the treatment of those outcomes that otherwise would have gone unnoticed. It can also lead to earlier detection of outcomes, at a less severe stage of the outcome, and thus potentially lower the cost associated with each of them [52].

Second, suppose a protocol mandates treatment of outcomes that is more intensive than the treatment that would have been provided in usual practice. This more intensive treatment can affect both the cost and effect associated with the outcomes. If the mandated treatment is itself cost-effective, its inclusion in the protocol will benefit the therapy that is associated with the larger number of outcomes because this therapy's relative cost and effect otherwise would have been less favorable than they are given the protocol-mandated services. If, on the other hand, the mandated treatment is not cost-effective, its inclusion in the protocol will disadvantage the therapy that is associated with the larger number of these outcomes because its relative cost and effect otherwise would have been more favorable than they are given the protocol-mandated services.

In the worst case, the protocol requires more aggressive active monitoring and treatment of outcomes than would occur in usual practice. In this case, it is difficult to determine how many outcomes would have been detected in usual practice, what the cost of care would have been, or whether the therapy tended to avoid the average outcome, those outcomes that in usual practice would never have been detected, or those outcomes that would have been most severe and caused the greatest harm in terms of cost and effect. As should be clear, in cases such as this, it is difficult if not impossible to correctly adjust for the impact of such protocol-induced services.

2.2.6. What should we do if the full benefit and cost of therapy are not expected to be observed during the period of observation in the trial?

Most trials that evaluate therapies for chronic conditions end study follow-up before the study medication would be discontinued in usual practice, the latter of which often occurs when the patient dies. In the cases where the trial ends follow-up earlier than when therapy would be discontinued, it is good practice to evaluate the cost and effect that were observed during the trial. In such a "within-trial" evaluation, we should maintain the same time horizons for cost and effect that were observed in the trial. For example, if follow-up for the trial was for 1 year, then cost and effect should be measured for 1 year.

For such trials, however, if long-term use yields outcomes that generally cannot be observed during the shorter timeframes employed in trials, or if the cost-effectiveness ratio is heterogeneous with time of follow-up, making therapeutic decisions based solely on results observed within short-term trials may be inappropriate. To address these limitations, a number of investigators have developed decision analytic models that use data from the trial and, in some cases, data from clinical registries and other sources, to attempt to address this issue [31,36,42]. (Note: As with the "within-trial" evaluation, we should maintain the same time horizons for the projections of cost and effect.) At a minimum, for trials that end follow-up before therapy would have ended, we need to make plans for credibly assessing longer term cost and effect.

One potential advantage of developing decision analytic models directly from trials with multiple years of follow-up is that we can evaluate the trajectory of the cost-effectiveness ratio over time. For example in a five-year trial, we can evaluate cost-effectiveness after each year of observation and then make projections for the first 5 years after the trial, the first 10, etc. Such a projection is provided in Table 2.1.

The table indicates that after 1 year, the therapy had not demonstrated value for the cost. As the period of follow-up within the trial increased, the evidence of value grew, although even after 5 years we could not rule out an upper limit for the confidence interval of the cost-effectiveness ratio of 123,000. Projection of results provides two important findings. First, at 5 years we have a reasonable approximation of the point estimate for the ratio that we project would be observed with longer follow-up. In other words, the ratio at 5 years is relatively homogeneous with projected results for longer periods of follow-up. Thus, we do not need to make a 40-year projection before we understand the likely point estimate for this therapy. Second, even after a relatively short projection, our results suggest that the confidence interval will narrow to a range where we can be confident of the value for the cost. Given the "model" uncertainty that surrounds 30- and 40-year projections, observing good value after only a short period of projection allows more confidence in our result.

Table 2.1 Cost-effectiveness evaluated for by years of follow-up within the trial and by projected years*

Years of follow-up	Point estimate	95% CI
Within the trial		
1	Dominated	168,884 to Dominated
2	282,857	45,577 to Dominated
3	73,529	Dominates to Dominated
4	12,074	Dominates to Dominated
5	15,258	Dominates to 122,772
Longer term projection		
10	12,246	Dominates to 42,263
15	8578	Dominates to 26,721
20	7320	681 to 21,841

*Authors' unpublished data.

Another advantage of developing a decision analytic model from the data from a trial is that the trial enables a limited assessment of the internal validity of the model. In other words, we are able to determine if the model can replicate the cost-effectiveness trajectory observed in the trial.

When it is inappropriate to perform an economic evaluation within a trial?

The presence or absence of an economic advantage should not be a deciding factor on whether to conduct an economic evaluation within a clinical trial, because both results provide useful information. Rather, as indicated in the section on naturalism of the trial, the most common reasons why it would be inappropriate to perform such an evaluation are when the trial design is such that no unbiased evidence about economic value will be observable (even nonsignificantly) during the period of observation. For example, if we have mandated so much care that we overwhelm all potential differences in cost, or if we have differentially followed participants based on outcome, it is unlikely that an economic assessment will be informative.

Practically, investigators may withhold performance of an economic evaluation if they believe that it will not affect the decision to use the therapy. For example, a therapy may be so effective that people will not worry about its cost, e.g., therapy that adds a year of life expectancy for a disease that is highly fatal and was previously untreatable. Similarly, in some health care systems, therapies may be so novel that clinicians will use them even if they are not cost effective.

What contributes to a successful economic evaluation within a trial?

Successful economic assessments conducted as part of clinical trials require a commitment to carry out such assessments. This commitment is characterized by early planning of the economic component of the trial, alerting the clinical investigators at the outset that the economic data will be collected along with the clinical data, and expecting all participants in the study to contribute both clinical and economic data to the study. In contrast, less successful economic assessments tend to have the clinical study designed independently and in advance of the economic study, the clinical investigators are recruited before the economic study is in place, and the economic study is introduced just as the trial initiates enrollment.

Trials least successful at recruiting participants are often ones in which the implicit message from the organizers is that the investigators are not obligated to enroll participants into the economic assessment. Trials should be designed so that enrolled participants are required to contribute both clinical and economic data to the study. Some may be concerned that such a requirement raises ethical issues, but trial exclusion criteria routinely eliminate patients who are unlikely to cooperate with data collection. We can minimize the chance that a patient believes she can participate in the trial and contribute clinical data but not economic data if we use a single informed consent agreement for both the clinical and economic information. If we seek to obtain billing data from providers who do not participate in the study, we should also ask study participants to sign forms that release their billing information.

Successful economic assessments as part of clinical trials also require cooperation and coordination among everyone involved in the trial, including the organizers, the clinical researchers, and the study participants. Disinterest or dissatisfaction among any of these groups can lead to collection of flawed data and can undermine the study. They also require a willingness to take the risk of determining that the therapy may be clinically effective yet not cost-effective.

Discussion

Many opportunities exist for the incorporation of economic assessments into the randomized trials used to assess medical therapies. When these assessments are conducted during the drug development process, they provide data about a drug's value early in its product life, and these data can be used by policy makers, drug manufacturers, health-care providers, and patients when the therapy is first introduced in the market. Better data about a therapy's economic effect potentially can be collected once it is used widely, but for making an early decision, data from phase III studies are the best that are available.

In this chapter, we have presented a broad overview of some of the current practices and methodologic issues that are part of an economic assessment. However, a wide diversity exists in the design and implementation of economic assessments. Some who organize economic assessments limit participation to study participants for whom large amounts of computerized billing data are available. Others focus on collecting hospitalization data in the form of electronic records from participating centers, thereby avoiding the need to deal with paper records. Another group of organizers prefers to collect the economic data from case report forms. This last option may be particularly useful for multinational trials, where the availability of electronic data may differ from country to country.

Economic analyses conducted within randomized trials share many design issues with traditional clinical trials, but they have unique issues as well.

Means for addressing the latter set of issues are undergoing rapid development, and the methods for doing these studies continue to evolve. We address a number of the latter issues in succeeding chapters.

References

1. Meltzer D. Accounting for future costs in medical cost-effectiveness analysis. *J Health Econ*. 1997; 16: 33–64.

2. Garber AM. Advances in cost-effectiveness of health interventions. In *Handbook of Health Economics Volume 1A*, edited by A.J. Culyer and J.P. Newhouse. Amsterdam: North-Holland, 2000.

3. Eisenberg JM. Clinical economics. A guide to the economic analysis of clinical practice. *JAMA*. 1989; 262: 2879–86.

4. Detsky AS, Naglie IG. A clinician's guide to cost-effectiveness analyis. *Ann Int Med*. 1990; 113: 147–54.

5. Gold MR, Siegel JE, Russell LB, Weinstein MC (eds). *Cost-Effectiveness in Health and Medicine*. Oxford: Oxford University Press, 1996.

6. Hornbrook MC. Definition and measurement of episodes of care in clinical and economic studies. In *Conference Proceedings: Cost Analysis Methodology for Clinical Practice Guidelines*, edited by M.C. Grady and K.A. Weis. DHHS Pub. No. (PHS)95-001. Rockville, MD: Agency for Health Care Policy and Research, 1995.

7. Keeler EB. Using Episodes of care in effectiveness research. In *Medical Effectiveness Research Data Methods*, edited by M.L. Grady and H.A. Schwartz. DHHS Pub. No (PHS) 92-0056. Rockville, MD: Agency for Health Care Policy and Research, 1992, pp. 161–72.

8. Steinwachs DM. Episode of care framework: utility for medical effectiveness research. In *Medical Effectiveness Research Data Methods*, edited by M.L. Grady and H.A. Schwartz. DHHS Pub. No (PHS) 92-0056. Rockville, MD: Agency for Health Care Policy and Research, 1992.

9. Hornbrook MC, Hurtado AV and Johnson RE. Health care episodes: definition, measurement, and use. *Medi Care Rev*. 1985; 42: 163–18.

10. Brainsky A, Glick H, Lydick E, Epstein R, Fox KM, Hawkes W, Kashner TM, Zimmerman ST, Magaziner J. The economic cost of hip fractures in community-dwelling older adults: a prospective study. *JAGS*. 1997; 45: 281–7.

11. Mehta SS, Suzuki S, Glick HA, Schulman KA. Determining an episode of care using claims data. Diabetic foot ulcer. *Diabetes Care* 1999; 22: 1110–15.

12. Schulman KA, Yabroff KR, Kong J, Gold KF, Rubenstein LE, Epstein AJ, Glick H. A claims data approach to defining an episode of care. *Health Services Research*. 1999; 34: 603–21.

13. Glick HA, Polsky D, Schulman K. Trial-based Economic Evaluations: An Overview of Design and Analysis. In *Economic Evaluation in Health Care. Merging Theory and Practice*, Chapter 6 edited by M. Drummond, A. McGuire, Oxford: Oxford University Press, 2001, pp. 113–40.

14. Glick H, Kinosian B, Schulman K. Decision analytic modelling: some uses in the evaluation of new pharmaceuticals. *Drug Inform J*. 1994; 28: 691–707.

15. Polsky DP, Glick HA, Willke R, Schulman K. Confidence intervals for cost-effectiveness ratios: a comparison of four methods. *Health Econ.* 1997; 6: 243–52.

16. Willan AR, O'Brien BJ. Confidence intervals for cost-effectiveness ratios: an application of Fieller's theorem. *Health Econ.* 1996; 5: 297–305.

17. Chaudhary MA, Stearns SC. Estimating confidence intervals for cost-effectiveness ratios: an example from a randomized trial. *Stat Med.* 1996; 15: 1447–58.

18. Hout BA van, Al MJ, Gordon GS, Rutten FFH. Costs, effects, and C/E ratios alongside a clinical trial. *Health Econ.* 1994; 3: 309–19.

19. O'Brien BJ, Drummond MF, Labelle RJ, Willan A. In search of power and significance: issues in the design and analysis of stochastic cost effectiveness studies in health care. *Med Care.* 1994; 32: 150–63.

20. Brown M, Glick HA, Harrell F, Herndon J, McCabe M, Moinpour C, Schulman KA, Smith T, Weeks J, Seils DM. Integrating economic analysis into cancer clinical trials: the National Cancer Institute - American Society of Clinical Oncology economics workbook. *Journal of the National Cancer Institute, Mongraphs.* 1988; (24), 1–28.

21. Towse A. What is NICE's threshold? An external view. Chapter 2. In *Cost Effectiveness Thresholds: Economic and Ethical Issues*, edited by N. Devlin, A. Towse, London: Kings Fund/Office for Health Economics, 2002.

22. Devlin N, Parkin D. Does NICE have a cost-effectiveness threshold and what other factors influence its decisions? A binary choice analysis. *Health Econ.* 2004; 13: 437–452.

23. George B, Harris A, Mitchell A. Cost-Effectiveness Analysis and the Consistency of Decision Making. Evidence from Pharmaceutical Reimbursement in Australia (1991 to 1996). *Pharmacoeconomics.* 2001; 19: 1103–9.

24. Hirth RA, Chernew ME, Miller E, Fendrick M, Weissert WG. Willingness to Pay for a Quality-Adjusted Life Year: In Search of a Standard, *Med Decision Making.* 2000; 20: 332–42.

25. Gupta AK. Pharmacoeconomic analysis of cicloprox nail lacquer solution 8% and the new oral antifungal agents used to treat dermatophyte toe onychomycosis in the United States. *J Am Acad Dermatol.* 2000; 43: S81–S95.

26. Cannell CF. A Summary of research studies of interviewing methodology, 1959-1970. vital and health statistics: series 2, Data Evaluation and Methods Research; Number 69, DHEW Publication; Number (HRA) 77–1343. Washington, D.C.: U.S. Government Printing Office, 1977.

27. Goossens ME, Rutten-van Molken MP, Vlaeyen JW, van der Linden SM. The cost diary: a method to measure direct and indirect costs in cost-effectiveness research. *J Clin Epi.* 2000; 53: 688–95.

28. Glick H, Willke R, Polsky D, Llana T, Alves WM, Kassell N, Schulman K. Economic analysis of tirilazad mesylate for aneurysmal subarachnoid hemorrhage: economic evaluation of a Phase III clinical trial in Europe and Australia. *Int J Tech Assess Health Care* 1998; 14: 145–60.

29. Legendre C, Norman D, Keating M, Maclaine G, Grant D. Valaciclovir prophylaxis of cytomegalovirus infection and disease in renal transplantation: an economic evaluation. *Transplantation* 2000; 70: 1463–8.

30. Schulman KA, Dorsainvil D, Yabroff KR, DiCesare J, Felser J, Eisenberg JM, Glick HA. Prospective economic evaluation accompanying a trial of GM-CSF/IL-3 in patients

undergoing autologous bone-marrow transplantation for hodgkin's and non-hodgkin's lymphoma. *Bone Marrow Transplant* 1998; 21: 607–14.

31. Mark DB, Hlatky MA, Califf RM, Naylor CD, Lee KL, Armstrong PW, Barbash G, White H, Simoons ML, Nelson CL. Cost effectiveness of thrombolytic therapy with tissue plasminogen activator as compared with streptokinase for acute myocardial infarction. *N Engl J Med*. 1995; 332: 1418–24.

32. Mauskopf J, Cates S, Griffin A, Neighbors D, Lamb S, Rutherford C. Cost effectiveness of zanamivir for the treatment of influenza in a high risk population in Australia. *Pharmacoeconomics*. 2000; 17: 611–20.

33. Markowitz M, Mauskopf J, Halpern M. Cost-effectiveness model of adjunctive lamotrogine for the treatment of epilepsy. *Neurology* 1998; 51: 1026–33.

34. Riviere M, Wang S, Leclerc C, Fitzsimon C, Tretiak R. Cost-effectiveness of simvastatin in the secondary prevention of coronary artery disease in Canada. *CMAJ*. 1997; 156: 991–97.

35. Johannesson M, Jonsson B, Kjekshus J, Olsson A, Pederson T, Wede H. Cost effective-ness of simvastatin treatment to lower cholesterol levels in patients with coronary heart disease. Scandinavian Simvastatin Study Group. *N Engl J Med*. 1997; 336: 332–6.

36. Glick H, Cook J, Kinosian B, Pitt B, Bourassa MG, Pouleur H, Gerth W. Costs and Effects of Enalapril Therapy in Patients with Symptomatic Heart Failure: An Economic Analysis of the Studies of Left Ventricular Dysfunction (SOLVD) Treatment Trial. *J Cardiac Fail*. 1995; 1: 371–80.

37. Mauskopf J, Richter A, Annemans L, Maclaine G. Cost-effectiveness model of cytomegalovirus management strategies in renal transplantation. Comparing valaciclovir prophylaxis with current practice. *Pharmacoeconomics* 2000; 18: 239–51.

38. Schulman KA, Buxton M, Glick H, Sculpher M, Guzman G, Kong J, Backhouse M, Mauskopf J, Bell L, Eisenberg JM. Results of the Economic Evaluation of the FIRST Study: A Multinational Prospective Economic Evaluation. *Int J Technol Assess Health Care*. 1996; 12: 698–713.

39. Glick HA, Orzol SM, Tooley JF, Remme WJ, Sasayama S, Pitt B. Economic evaluation of the Randomized Aldactone Evaluation Study (RALES): treatment of patients with severe heart failure. *Cardiovasc Drugs Therapy* 2002; 16: 53–9.

40. Department of Health and Human Services, Health Care Financing Administration. Medicare program: hospital inpatient prospective payment systems. *Federal Register*. August, 1991; 56: 4821.

41. Department of Health and Human Services, Health Care Financing Administration. Medicare program: fee schedule for physicians' services: final rule. *Federal Register*. (Addendum B) November 25, 1991; 56: 59502–811.

42. Hsiao WC, Braun P, Dunn DL, Becker ER, Yntema D, Verrilli DK, Stamenovic E, Chen SP. An overview of the development and refinement of the resource-based rela-tive value scale. *Med Care* 1992; 30(suppl): NS1-NS12.

43. Schulman K, Burke J, Drummond M, Davies L, Carlsson P, Gruger J, Harris A, Lucioni C, Gisbert R, Llana T, Tom E, Bloom B, Willke R, Glick H. Resource costing for multina-tional neurologic clinical trials: methods and results. *Health Econ*. 1998; 7: 629–38.

44. Bridges M, Jacobs P. Obtaining estimates of marginal cost by DRG. *Healthcare Financial Management*. 1986; 10: 40–6.

45. Granneman TW, Brown RS, Pauly MV. Estimating hospital costs. A multiple-output analysis. *J Health Econ.* 1986; 5: 107–27.

46. Finkler SA. Cost finding for high-technology, high-cost services: current practice and a possible alternative. *Health Care Manage Rev.* 1980; 5: 17–29.

47. Bauer MS, Williford WO, Dawson EE, Akiskal HS, Altshuler L, Fye C, Gelenberg A, Glick H, Kinosian B, Sajatovic M. Principles of effectiveness trials and their implementation in VA Cooperative Study #430: 'Reducing the efficacy-effectiveness gap in bipolar disorder'. *J Affect Disord.* 2001; 67: 61–78.

48. Polsky D, Doshi JA, Bauer MS, Glick HA. Clinical Trial-Based Cost-Effectiveness Analyses of Antipsychotics. *Am J Psychiatry* In press.

49. The SOLVD Investigators. Effect of enalapril on survival in patients with reduced left ventricular ejection fractions and congestive heart failure. *NEJM.* 1991; 325: 293–302.

50. Scandinavian Simvastatin Survival Study Group. Randomised trial of cholesterol lowering in 4444 patients with coronary heart disease: the Scandinavian Simvastatin Survival Study (4S). *Lancet* 1994; 344: 1383–9.

51. Rubin DB. Inference and missing data. *Biometrika* 1976; 63: 581–92.

52. Eisenberg JM, Glick H, Koffer H. Pharmacoeconomics: economic evaluation of pharmaceuticals. Chapter 24 in *Pharmacoepidemiology.* edited by B Strom. New York: Churchill Livingstone, 1989. Pages 325–50.

Chapter 3

Valuing medical service use

As indicated in Chapter 2, in most trials, investigators measure medical service use in study case report forms. Once we have collected information about medical service use, we need to translate this use into a cost that can be compared with the measure of study effectiveness. Commonly this translation is done by identifying price weights independently from particular participants' experiences and multiplying medical service use by price weights for those services. The issues related to selection of an appropriate set of price weights are the main focus of the current chapter.

An alternative strategy, in which we use the case report form to record the cost of services used, is rarely, if ever, adopted because those who record information in case report forms often are not aware of the cost associated with medical service use, in part because cost information may not be readily available. In addition, discrepancies between health care charge and actual cost are widespread in the United States [1] and possibly in other countries. Those collecting the data may not be sufficiently familiar with economic principles to determine whether the price data they might obtain are adequate proxies for economic cost.

A third alternative occurs in trials that are conducted in health systems that have ready access to administrative data such as billing records. In these studies, we may be able to use these systems to obtain measures of both medical service use and cost (or expenditure). In this chapter, we briefly discuss the strengths and potential weaknesses of the use of these data.

Finally, trials often either enroll or follow participants over a period of several years. We thus discuss adjusting for inflation and time preference so that the resulting cost (and effect) from different years can be compared.

No matter which strategy for costing we choose for the valuation of medical service use, appropriate price weights depend on the study's perspective. From a social perspective, price weights should reflect social opportunity cost, which need not equal payment. From other perspectives, it may be more appropriate for price weights to reflect payment. From all perspectives, price weights should reflect marginal not average cost. Particularly from the social perspective, it is rare that investigators can identify measures of social opportunity cost. The common solution is to develop second-best approximations of this cost. Most of the discussion in this chapter relates to these second-best approximations.

3.1. **Price weights**

As we have indicated, one strategy for developing the cost outcome for the trial is to measure medical service use and value it by use of price weights. In this section, we discuss common sources of these price weights, their strengths and weaknesses, and practical issues related to their collection and use.

3.1.1. **National and center-specific price weights**

Wherever they are available, national tariffs, for example, diagnosis-related group (DRG) payments in Australia or the United States or health resource group (HRG) payments in Great Britain, are a commonly used and well-accepted source of price weights for costing out medical service use. Their advantages include that they usually provide price weights for most if not all of the services that are measured in the trial; they are inexpensive to obtain; within individual countries, they are usually developed by use of a common methodology; and they make it difficult for investigators to pick and choose among price weights to make an intervention look more or less favorable than it should. The fact that these tariffs represent what is spent by governments may also be considered an advantage, particularly by governmental decision-making bodies.

Center-specific price weights, which are often obtained from the institutions in which the trial was conducted, but in some data-poor environments, are obtained from any institution in a country for which the data are available, are another commonly used source of price weights for costing out medical service use. One of the primary advantages of center-specific price weights is that they provide a more accurate estimate of the cost that was actually incurred within the trial. In addition, as will be shown later in this chapter in Box 3.2, cost and medical service use can have important interactions that, if not accounted for, can lead to biased results. Given that efficient producers use greater amounts of relatively less costly services and smaller amounts of relatively more costly services, use of a single set of price weights for all providers will tend to overstate cost. This principle holds for studies performed in a single center, in multiple centers in a single country, or in multiple centers in multiple countries.

While the most appropriate source of price weights may depend on whether the question we are asking is more national or center specific, the question being asked cannot be our only consideration when we choose an appropriate set of price weights. For example, if our goal is to make national resource allocation decisions – in which case the national cost implications of a therapy are most relevant – we might conclude that use of a set of national price weights would yield data appropriate for making such decisions. However, the representativeness of the resulting cost estimates depends on the representativeness of both medical service use and price weights. Once one factor is unrepresentative – for example, if medical service use is measured in an unrepresentative set of centers – it is an open question whether ensuring that the other factor is representative necessarily yields the best estimates. While it is easy for us to recommend that you assess the sensitivity of your results to the source of price weights – by having you use center-specific and national sources for these weights – we also recognize that such a strategy is costly. If you decide to use only one set of price weights, you should weigh the issues of representativeness and bias when making your selection.

3.1.2. Accuracy of national tariffs

Some authors have raised concerns that national tariffs do not equal cost. For example, Beck et al. [2] compared British Trust tariffs with the results of a service-specific costing exercise. They found substantial differences between the two, with differences increasing as the intensity of services increased. Heerey et al. [3] compared results from microcosting versus Irish DRGs and found differences ranging between –9 and 66%. Shwartz et al. [4] compared estimates of cost derived by multiplying U.S. charges times Federal cost-to-charge ratios with estimates of cost derived by use of relative value units. They concluded that at the patient level the charge-adjusted estimates were inaccurate, but that the average of the charge-adjusted estimates across groups of patients was usually within 10% of the relative value estimates.

Some of these differences may have occurred simply because cost differs by center, in which case national tariffs need not agree with the cost in any single center. Others may have more to do with differences in the level of aggregation that are employed by the different data sources than they do with the fact that some estimates are national and some are local. For example, had Beck et al. compared service-specific costing to costing based on center-specific average cost per day, they might have seen similar kinds of differences, particularly for the cost gradient between different levels of patient severity.

Whether or not national tariffs are accurate, the more important question is whether these differences are likely to affect the conclusions of economic analyses? Common sense suggests they should, and Rittenhouse et al. [5] and Reed et al. [6] have argued that they may. However, there is at best limited evidence about whether or not they do. In two studies that examined this issue, both Chumney *et al.* [7] and Taira *et al.* [8] found that costing method affected the estimate of cost by treatment group. However, in both cases, the intervention was effective enough that the authors concluded that the differences did not lead to conflicting recommendations about adoption.

3.1.3. **Incomplete sets of price weights**

In many trials, price weights are derived from a selected set of centers that participated in the trial. As Goeree *et al.* have reported, the number of centers from which price weights are derived may affect the results of the study [9]. The analog in multinational trials is that price weights are often collected from a subset of countries that participated in the trial. Within each country, they are often derived from a single source, which in the same trial can vary between center-specific price weights in some countries to national tariffs in others. The countries from which price weights are collected might be ones that: enroll a large number of participants in the trial; represent the spectrum of economic development among countries that participated in the trial; have readily available price weights; or have regulators that require a submission for reimbursement. In industry-sponsored studies, they also may include countries in which the study sponsor wishes to make economic claims.

Eventually, we need to obtain price weights for every service we intend to cost out in our analysis. However, it may be costly to obtain weights for all services in all centers and countries that participated in the trial. When we sample price weights, the medical services for which price weights are collected, for example, hospital cost by diagnosis, outpatient visits, and days in long-term care facilities, might be those observed most frequently in the trial, those that are considered likely to be affected by the intervention, or – if we use an imputation procedure to estimate price weights for some medical services – those that have particularly high or low price weights.

When we collect price weights for a subset of the medical services that have been observed in a trial, we must develop a method for imputing price weights for the remaining services. If little or no additional information is available about these services, we may want to use the mean price weight for similar services. For example, for hospitalization, we might use the simple average of the price weight estimates from hospitalizations for which these estimates are available.

If additional information is available, such as relative values for a medical service – for example, U.S. or Australian DRG weights, British HRG weights, or the U.S. physician fee schedule – a prediction model can be developed that uses the available price weight estimates as the outcome variable, and the relative values and variables representing the countries as the explanatory variables [10,11].

If we can build such a prediction model, one question that may arise has to do with the number of countries in which we should collect price weights and the number of price weights we should collect within each country. Based on simulation, Glick *et al.* [11] have reported that imputation error is minimized when we obtain estimates for fewer types of services from as many countries as feasible, rather than by obtaining estimates for more types of services in fewer countries. However, reduction of imputation error may need to be traded-off against the cost of data collection. In our experience, the cost of initiation of data collection in an additional country usually far exceeds the cost of obtaining an equivalent number of additional price weight estimates in countries where these data are already being collected.

3.1.4. **Sources of price weights**

Sources of price weights that represent proxies for cost differ by country and by medical service. For inpatient services, many countries now use patient classification systems like DRGs or HRGs. Some of these systems provide measures of both the relative cost of a hospital stay – a relative value or a relative weight – and the reimbursement/cost for a stay; others provide measures of relative cost, and we must then independently identify the cost per relative weight. Examples of these weights are provided in Table 3.1. For international studies, particularly those enrolling participants in the developing world, The WHO has developed estimates of price weights for inpatient care in at least 49 countries [12].

The U.S. has a number of sources of data on outpatient fees, as does the U.K. For the U.S., these include the Medicare Fee Schedule (http://www.cms.hhs.gov/physicianfeesched/pfsrvf/list.asp?), the Clinical Diagnostic Laboratory Fee Schedule (http://new.cms.hhs.gov/ClinicalLabFeeSched/02_clinlab.asp#TopOfPage), and the Medicare Durable Good Fee Schedule (http://new.cms.hhs.gov/DMEPOSFeeSched/LSDMEPOSFEE/list.asp#TopOfPage). In the U.K., they include NHS Reference Costs (see web address in Table 3.1) which give average cost and dispersion statistics for first and subsequent outpatient attendances, by HRG and specialty. See Table 3.2 for examples of these data from the U.S.

For medication costs, the most common practice in the U.S. has been to use the average wholesale price (AWP), the price paid by wholesalers to manufacturers, which can be obtained from various commercially available publications. In other countries such as the U.K., the drug prices are generally obtained from national formulary lists [13]. Pauly [14] has recently criticized the use of measures such as AWP for studies that adopt a societal perspective because AWP often overstates the marginal cost of drugs. His work provides a detailed overview of the issues and concerns.

Table 3.1 Comparative diagnosis-related group (DRG) weights and average lengths of stay from Australia, Great Britain, and the United States*

Diagnosis/procedure	Australia				U.K.				U.S.		
	DRG	Relative weight	ALOS†	Cost ($A)	HRG	Relative weight	ALOS	Cost (£UK)	DRG	Relative weight	ALOS
Chest pain	F74Z	0.42	1.54	1296	E36	0.258352	2.3	580	143	0.57	2.1
Cholecystectomy w/common bile duct exploration, no cc	H07B	2.47	5.77	7698	G14	1.175847	4.7	2640	196	1.60	5.7
GI hemorrhage w/cc	G61A	0.79	3.49	2476	F64	0.449889	4.2	1010	174	1.01	4.7
GI obstruction w/cc	G65A	1.54	5.96	4789	P12	0.769265	3.5	1727	180	0.98	5.4
Heart failure and shock	F64Z	1.20	5.40	3736	E18	0.715367	7.3	1606	127	1.03	5.2
Hernia (< 10 yr, AU; < 17 yr U.S.)	G10Z	0.84	1.33	2618	F73	0.664588	2.1	1492	163	0.67	2.9
Liver transplant	A01Z	26.57	29.27	82885	G01	8.220045	13.2	18454	480	8.94	17.9

*Sources: Australia, Round 8 public sector weights, http://www.health.gov.au/internet/wcms/publishing.nsf/Content/health-casemix-costing-fc_r8; U.K., 2005 National Reference Costs, http://www.dh.gov.uk/PolicyAndGuidance/OrganisationPolicy/FinanceAndPlanning/NHSReferenceCosts/fs/en; U.S., 2006 DRG relative weights, http://www.cms.hhs.gov/acuteinpatientpps/ffd/itemdetail.asp?filterType=none&filterByDID=99&sortByDID=2&sortOrder=ascending&itemID=CMS022585. U.S. Medicare relative weights omit surgical and attending physician fees, which are paid for separately by use of the Medicare fee schedule.

†ALOS = average length of stay; cc = comorbid conditions; yr = years

Table 3.2 Cost of selected outpatient services in the U.S.[†]

Medicare Fee Schedule ($2004)

Service	Non-facility fee (RVU * $37.34)
Office visit, new	
Problem focused history and examination; straight forward medical decision making; typically spend 10 min face-to-face	36
Detailed history and examination; medical decision making of low complexity; typically spend 30 min face-to-face	96
Comprehensive history and examination; medical decision making of high complexity; typically spend 60 min face-to-face	172

Clinical Diagnostic Laboratory Fee Schedule ($2003)

Service	National midpoint
Heparin assay	24.72
Blood platelet aggregation	40.56
Prothrombin time	7.42

Medicare Durable Good Fee Schedule ($2004)

Service	Average of floor and ceiling costs
Drug infusion pump supplies	43.02
Glucose monitor platforms	3.79
Rose-tinted glasses	9.28

[†]See web addresses, p. 39. RVU = relative value unit

If neither national nor local price weights are readily available, we may use price weights derived from more detailed costing studies. For example, the Dutch Health Insurance Board, with the approval of the Minister of Public Health, Welfare and Sport have issued guidelines for standardizing the estimation of price weights [15,16]. Other examples of these more detailed costing studies include those for general hospital cost by Garattini *et al.* [17] and Oostenbrink *et al.* [18] or hospital pharmacy cost by Scullen *et al.* [19]. Alternatively, it may be possible to develop trial-specific costing exercises, for example by analysis of accounting data [20], use of the top-down cost-block program [21,22], estimation of hospital cost functions [23–25], or time and motion studies [26] (see Box 3.1).

Box 3.1 Time and motion studies

A number of methods can be used to assess the time that health professionals spend providing care, and with that, its cost. These include time and motion, work or activity sampling, logging, and historical averaging [26–29]. These methods may entail observer ratings, remote beeper-prompted recording, or self-reporting. Each method has its strengths and weaknesses, including accuracy, cost, convenience, and artifacts of observation/observability (see Oddone *et al.* [28] and Pelletier *et al.* [29] for reviews of these methods).

One of the most common methods is the time and motion study. Steps in conducting a time and motion study include first, enumeration of the services provided by identifying and defining each activity. This activity is sometimes referred to as determining the exact production process [26]. Second, we define a time standard for each service by observer measurement, self measurement, or self estimation via recall. Third, we define a measure of frequency for each service. Fourth, we identify the supplies and equipments utilized by each service. Fifth, we identify the fixed and variable costs by service

In a recent study, Glick *et al.* [30] used a provider self-report study design to estimate the time spent by psychiatric clinical nurse specialist care managers for clinic visits made by patients with bipolar disorder. Figure B3.1.1 reports the results of this analysis. Open circles represent the average of observed minutes per visit, stratified by the number of visits per day; the solid line represents predicted minutes per visit. Average time per clinic visit was 33.5 min (data not shown). Depending on the number of visits in a day, however, it ranged from approximately 35 min per visit when there were 1–4 visits per day to approximately 10–15 min per day, when there were 14 or more visits per day. If we plan an intervention that will substantially change the number of visits per day, these data provide an indication about how cost – and effectiveness? – might change if the intervention is not accompanied by changes in staffing patterns.

Time and motion methodologic issues

When we are planning to conduct a time and motion study, there are a number of methodologic issues we should consider, having to do with sample size, variability among patients, and a set of issues related to identifying boundaries between measured activities.

Sample size estimation: Sample size estimation for time and motion estimates is often based on the desired precision of the mean of our time estimates. If we are primarily interested in the mean time for an activity,

Box 3.1 Time and motion studies *(continued)*

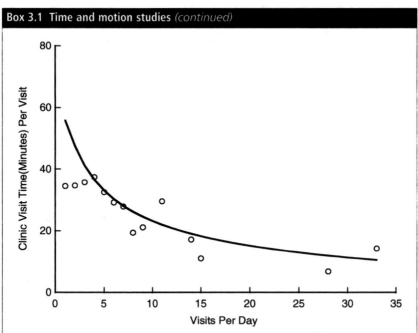

Fig. 3.1.1 Graph of observed (open circles) and predicted (solid line) average minutes of clinic visit time per clinic visit, stratified by the number of visits per day. Source: Glick *et al.* [30].
Reproduced from Glick HA, Kinosian B, McBride L, Williford WO, Bauer MS. Clinical nurse specialist care manager's time commitments in a disease management programme for bipolar disorder. *Bipolar Disorders*, 2004: 6:452-59 with permission from Blackwell Publishing.

we estimate a sample size to ensure a confidence interval of a specified length around a mean or set of means. If we are primarily interested in determining whether the mean for one activity differs from that of another, we estimate a sample size for a difference in means. The two formulas follow:

$$\text{Sample size for a mean: } n = \left(\frac{z_\alpha \text{SD}}{w} \right)$$

$$\text{Sample size for a difference in means: } n = \left(\frac{2\text{SD}^2 (z_\alpha + z_\beta)^2}{\Delta^2} \right),$$

where n equals the sample size for the measurement; z_α is the z score for the α error (commonly 1.96); SD equals the standard deviation; w is the width of the half interval (e.g., if the mean is 5 min and our goal is to observe a

Box 3.1 Time and motion studies *(continued)*

confidence interval ranging from 4 to 6 min, $w = 1$); z_β = the z score for the β error (commonly 0.84); and Δ equals the difference in mean times.

If the number of providers and patients is limited, and we are making multiple observations on both providers and patients, we may want to account for the lack of independence between measurements. To do so, we would use sample size formulas for two-stage cluster sampling.

Accounting for patient variability: Time, and thus cost, may vary across different types of patients. In one study, Iglar defined time standards for seven different patient types [31].

Identifying boundaries between activities: Although it may be easy to conceptually define boundaries between different activities, in practice different observers may disagree about when one activity has stopped and another has started. One approach to addressing this issue is to have multiple observers watch the same provider–patient diad.

Starting and stopping an activity: While conceptualization of the production process may generally assume that it is linear, i.e. one starts the task and continues until one completes it, in practice, this process is often interrupted. We should develop rules for how we count time when the process is interrupted.

Joint time: Another common assumption about the production process is that providers perform a single activity at a time. However, a nurse might enter a patient's room, place an automated blood pressure cuff on the patient's arm, take the patient's temperature, enter notes in the patients' chart, and finally obtain a reading of the patient's blood pressure. Allocation of time to each of these individual activities is arbitrary. While some analysts may adopt accounting procedures and allocate it by dividing it up between the activities that were performed – for example by dividing observed time equally between the shared activities – from an economic perspective, the marginal time for each activity depends in part on how the length of the encounter would have changed had the nurse performed some but not others of the activity.

Work sampling

As an alternative to time and motion techniques, in which people are observed, or are self-timed performing a sequence of activities, some authors have argued that work sampling is a superior technique [28]. In work sampling, data are recorded about what providers are doing at particular times in the day. For example, we can determine how a nurse allocates her time doing a number of different activities by identifying exactly what he was doing at 40 different times during the day.

Box 3.1 Time and motion studies *(continued)*

For example, in one study, "A small, portable random alarm beeper (JD-7, Divilbliss Electronics, Champaign, IL) was utilized to determine the sampled time points. The beeper was set at a predetermined frequency (5.0/h); beeps occurred at random so that the [depression clinical specialists] DCSs could not anticipate the sample time point .... At each beep, the DCS recorded what they were doing (activity) and with whom (contact) on a code form they carried with them on a clipboard" [32]. Table B3.1.1 shows the principal results from a work sampling study.

Of note, this technique does not eliminate problems such as joint time, given that the provider may be performing multiple activities at the time when they are asked to record what they are doing.

Table B3.1.1 Research nurse's work activities

Work activity	Mean proportion of workday (95% CI)
Research related	
Screening patients	10.2 (7.9–12.5)
Completing forms	11.2 (7.1–15.4)
Computer	4.1 (2.4–5.9)
Phone, research*	0.8 (0.3–1.3)
Other	16.2 (11.7–20.7)
Subtotal	42.5 (38.1–46.7)
Patient care	
Discussing patient care	9.7 (6.4–13.0)
Providing education	4.4 (3.4–5.4)
On phone with patient*	2.5 (1.4–3.5)
Phone, other patient care*	1.7 (0.8–2.6)
Computer	4.3 (2.2–6.4)
Other	6.2 (3.0–9.4)
Subtotal	28.8 (24.1–33.2)
Personal	16.4 (12.0–20.7)
In transit	12.5 (9.1–15.9)
Total	100.2†

*"Phone, research": research assistant or study coordinating center listed as contact; "On phone with patient": patient listed as contact; "Phone, other patient care": all other phone observations.

†Total is greater than 100% due to rounding error.

Oddone et al., [28]

Reproduced from Oddone E. Weinberger M. Hurder A. Henderson W. Simel D. Measuring activities in clinical trials using random work sampling: implications for cost-effectiveness analysis and measurement of the intervention. *Journal of Clinical Epidemiology* 1995; 48: 1011-18 with permission from Elsevier.

3.1.5. **Comparability of price weights from multiple countries**

As Schulman *et al.* [10] have pointed out, if we collect price weights from multiple countries, the resulting estimates may not be directly comparable. One source of this lack of comparability may be that the resource intensity associated with a service in one country, for example, a day in the intensive care unit (ICU), may differ from the resource intensity of a similarly labeled service in another country (e.g., the staff to patient ratio or training of staff in ICUs may differ across countries). Another source of this lack of comparability may be variation in countries' handling of the cost of capital. For example, in some countries it may be included in hospital budgets; in others it may be included in public budgets. Lack of comparability may also arise because of variation in countries' accounting standards and practices, etc.

This heterogeneity in price weights may lead to problems of transferability of the study results. It should not bias the pooled result of the evaluation, however, so long as we multiply country-specific measures of medical service use times country-specific price weights. On the other hand, we may want to adjust the observed price weights to make them comparable between countries.

One set of modifications may include trying to equate the methods different countries use to account for capital expenditure and overhead. For example, in their costing exercise, Schulman *et al.* attempted to remove overhead and capital costs when they were present in the price weights [10]. Another set of modifications has to do with translating all price weights into a common currency. This latter conversion is usually accomplished by use of purchasing power parity statistics [33] (see Table 3.3). Purchasing power parities are currency conversion factors that eliminate differences in price levels between countries. Conversion using purchasing power parity is preferred over use of exchange rates because the former provides a comparative measure of the buying power of a currency rather than a reflection of the supply of currency in international markets [34].

3.1.6. **Use of country-specific price weights or averaging price weights among countries**

When we have price weight data from more than one country, we also need to decide whether to apply country-specific price weights to medical service use observed in that country or whether to average the price weights from all study centers into a single set of price weights. Rationales for such averaging may include (1) that by reducing the variance associated with different prices in different countries, we may reduce the overall variance in the cost outcome and (2) that results based on an average set of price weight estimates might be

Table 3.3 Selected 2005 purchasing power parities*

Country	Purchasing power parity
Australia	1.38
Canada	1.25
Czech Republic	14.2
France	0.902
Germany	0.913
Hungary	126
Italy	0.85
Japan	129
Mexico	7.37
Netherlands	0.899
Spain	0.765
Sweden	9.06
Switzerland	1.68
United Kingdom	0.627
United States	1.00

*Source: Organization for Economic Cooperation and Development. Main economic indicators, March 2006. http://www.oecd.org/dataoecd/61/54/18598754.pdf

more representative. The validity of this latter rationale is unclear, given that it is possible that no individual country makes purchasing/production decisions based on the averaged price weights.

Notwithstanding these rationales, because relative prices can affect quantities of services provided, and because in the face of variations in practice, the treatment's effect on medical service use and outcome can differ, whenever feasible, we should multiply country-specific price weight estimates times country-specific quantities. In other words, we should not use an averaged set of price weight estimates. This practice will avoid potential biases that can arise due to substitution effects in different countries [35]; in some cases, it may also appropriately increase the variance in the cost outcome that is being evaluated. (See Box 3.2.)

For countries for which price weight data are not available, ideally, we should use price weight estimates from similar countries. For example, internationally, we might use price weights from other countries that have similar health care expenditure data as documented by agencies such as the Organisation for Economic Co-operation and Development [36]. Alternately, within a country,

Box 3.2 Substitution effects and averaging of price weight estimates

Should we multiply center-specific quantities times center-specific price weight estimates? Or alternatively, should we multiply these quantities times a single set of price weights that represents the average of the price weights from all study centers? The following example indicates the potential problems that can arise from the latter strategy.

Assume that you are conducting a trial in two centers. In center 1, the relative cost of a day in an ICU care compared with a day in a routine care unit is high and in center 2, the relative cost of a day in the ICU is low. Assume that institutions respond to these differences in relative cost, and more care in the ICU is used in center 2 with its lower relative cost of ICU. In this case, we would expect that use of the average of the prices from the two centers to evaluate all medical service use in the trial would lead to a biased result.

Table B3.2.1 provides hypothetical data on length of stay for the four patients who are enrolled in the trial (two in treatment group 1 and two in treatment group 2). As indicated in the assumptions above, patients treated in center 2 remain longer in the ICU and shorter in routine care units than do those treated in center 1.

Table B3.2.2 shows the hypothetical center-specific price weights (column 1). The observed differences in cost are meant to represent differences in the relative price of inputs or in the relative intensity of services that are being provided in what is being called ICU and routine care units. They are not meant to reflect differences in pricing strategies that are unrelated to input prices or intensity of service.

The table also shows several potential averages of the price weights that might instead be used to value medical service use of individuals in the trial. These include the simple average (column 2). For example, the ICU estimate of 750 was calculated as follows: (1000 + 500)/2. They also include a weighted average, with weights based on the center-specific total number of days in each unit (column 3). For example, the ICU estimate of

Table B3.2.1 Data on average length of stay

	Center 1		Center 2	
	Treatment		Treatment	
Unit	1	2	1	2
ICU	3	3	8	4
Routine	16	8	10	6

Box 3.2 Substitution effects and averaging of price weight estimates *(continued)*

Table B3.2.2 Price weight data

Medical service	Center-specific	Simple average	Weighted average	Treatment-specific weighted average	
				1	2
Center 1					
ICU	1000	750	667	636	714
Routine	250	325	310	308	314
Center 2					
ICU	500	750	667	636	714
Routine	400	325	310	308	314

667 was calculated as follows: $([1000 \times 6] + [500 \times 12])/18$. Finally, a third possibility is a set of treatment-specific weighted average price weight estimates, in which separate weighted average price weight estimates are derived for each treatment group (columns 4 and 5). For example, the 636 estimate of ICU cost for treatment group 1 was calculated as follows: $([1000 \times 3]+[500 \times 8])/11$.

Table B3.2.3 shows the treatment-group-specific estimates of mean and standard deviation for hospital cost derived using the different price weight estimation strategies. Using the center-specific data, the means ±SD for treatment groups 1 and 2 were 7500 (707) and 4700 (424), respectively. The difference was 2800 (SE, 583).

Use of the simple average of the price weights yielded estimates of the means and differences that were all greater than those that were estimated using the center-specific data (e.g., a mean difference of 3450, SE, 901). Use of weighted average price weights yielded a higher estimate of mean cost

Table B3.2.3 Estimated means and standard deviations derived using the four sets of price weight estimates

Price weight Estimate	Treatment 1		Treatment 2		Difference	
	Mean	SD	Mean	SD	Mean	SE
Center-specific	7500	707	4700	424	2800	583
Simple average	8350	1273	4900	71	3450	901
Weighted average	7697	1042	4503	33	3193	737
Treatment-specific weighted average	7500	944	4700	61	2800	669

Box 3.2 Substitution effects and averaging of price weight estimates *(continued)*

for those in treatment group 1, a lower estimate for those in treatment group 2, a higher estimate of the incremental cost (e.g., a mean difference of 3193, SE, 737). Finally, use of the treatment-specific weighted average price weights yielded point estimates that were the same as those derived using center-specific price weights (i.e., by definition use of these weights leaves the univariate estimate of incremental cost unchanged); however, even in this case, use of an averaged set of price weights led to mixed results for the standard deviations in the point estimates, and a larger standard error for the difference in costs (669).

Thus, in the example, use of averaged price weight estimates generally led to biased estimates of the treatments' effects on cost, and there was no consistent reduction in the standard deviations of the estimates (i.e., one of the purported reasons for using averaged price weight estimates).

In actual practice, when we calculate cost by multiplying estimates of medical service use times center-specific price weight estimates, the results can be affected by both substitution and income effects (i.e., more well-to-do centers may buy more of all services, whereas less well-to-do centers may buy fewer of all services). In two trials that we have analyzed (unpublished data), we found less consistency in the direction of the impacts of the use of center-specific versus averaged price weight estimates than would be suggested by the example above. While in some instances the estimates of incremental cost were biased upwards, there were also instances where they were biased downwards. In addition, in some cases, the standard deviations that resulted from the use of pooled price weight estimates were lower than those that resulted from using center-specific price weight estimate.

There are good theoretical reasons to multiply center-specific price weight estimates times center-specific medical service use [35]. While use of pooled price weight estimates may reduce variance in the resulting cost estimate, it may also increase it. Also, given that price weights may affect practice, and that the average practice reflected in the trial is unlikely to reflect practice in any other set of specific centers, it is unclear that use of an averaged set of price weights makes the results more representative.

Source: Reproduced from Glick HA, Polsky D, Schulman K. Trial-Based Economic Evaluations: An Overview of Design and Analysis. Chapter 6 in Drummond M, McGuire A (eds.) Economic Evaluation in Health Care Merging Theory and Practice, Oxford University Press, 2001, 113–40 by permission of Oxford University Press.

if we are missing price weights from an academic medical center, we might use price weights from other academic medical centers in their stead. Practically, however, many investigators have used a single set of price weights reflecting the average of the available price weights [10].

3.2. **Program cost**

Some trials, for example those evaluating novel behavioral interventions, assess programs that provide bundles of services that may not have price weights associated with them. In these cases, there is a need to evaluate the cost of these programs and to assess how this cost changes as the number of participants changes.

In some cases, researchers have developed general instruments that are meant for use in costing programs of a certain type, such as the Drug Abuse Treatment Cost Analysis Program (DATCAP) [37] and the Brief DATCAP [38]. The DATCAP captures the cost of personnel (direct salaries, fringe benefits, and volunteers), supplies and materials (medical, office, housekeeping, and food), major equipments (office furniture, computers, electronics, medical, and residential), contracted services (laboratory, repairs/maintenance, security, housekeeping, and advertising), buildings and facilities (total space, total usable space, rate of use, and rental rate), miscellaneous resources (utilities, insurance, taxes, telephone, and printing), and those not recorded elsewhere (goods, services, and contracts) [37]. Various members of the treatment program's staff, such as administrators, therapist coordinators, and accounting/finance personnel, are asked to identify specific services, and cost data are usually collected from general ledgers, personnel reports, expenditure reports, and inventory reports.

Other researchers have implemented time analyses (see Box 3.1). For example, Anderson *et al.* developed site-specific diaries for the identification of cost by type of service and day of the week and asked all staff members who provided any of 94 different treatment and nontreatment services to track cost over the course of 1 week [39]. The staff indicated the amount of time and materials used in providing these services during each day of the week. Barrett *et al.*, on the other hand, used data from patient files and electronic databases in their development of the Secure Facilities Service Use Schedule [40].

In other cases, researchers have developed trial-specific instruments designed to evaluate the cost of the programs evaluated in the trials. For example, in the Diabetes Prevention Program (DPP), investigators asked DPP staff members to respond to questionnaires that elicited information about the types of personnel that participated in the intervention; the amount of time they participated; the health education materials distributed; and the like [41]. In the A Stop Smoking In Schools Trial (ASSIST), investigators asked ASSIST staff to respond weekly to standardized forms that asked about staff time, travel time and distance, consumables, accommodation, and vouchers for peer supporters who implemented the intervention [42]. Finally, in the Hartslag Limburg community heart health intervention, investigators followed a 3-step approach in which they (1) identified the components of the intervention that would be included in the costing; (2) identified the methods that would be used to determine the material and personnel resources needed for implementing these components; and (3) valued the material and personnel [43].

Although methods like those above can be used to evaluate either marginal or average cost, as described, many of these investigators and their instruments quantified average rather than marginal cost.

3.3. **Administrative data**

Finally, in some cases, study participants are treated in health care systems that maintain administrative databases that quantify either medical service use, cost/payment, or both service use and cost/payment for patients in the trial. Examples in the U.S. include U.S. Medicare records, U.S. Veterans Administration (VA) records, and health maintenance organization records. If it is possible for investigators to obtain access to these data, they may be used to quantify the cost of care provided in the trial.

Advantages of use of such records include that they usually capture service use independent of site of care; and they are independent of fallible participant recall. At the same time, use of these databases may raise potential problems that should be solved if they are to provide accurate measures of cost in a timely fashion. Due to their idiosyncrasies and complexities, it is difficult if not impossible to give specific advice about the use of any single administrative database. Rather, we identify general issues that investigators should consider when they evaluate use of such databases.

First, some administrative databases aggregate service use. For example, they may provide an estimate of the total cost or charge for a hospitalization even if it lasts for weeks or months. Alternatively, physicians may combine several visits in a single bill, etc. Given that investigators need to distinguish the cost that is incurred prior to randomization, from randomization until the end of follow-up, and after the end of follow-up, we must ensure that the potential database allows disaggregation of this aggregated cost, or that it at least allows for the allocation of this cost to the different time periods. For example, if a participant is randomized on the fifth day of a 10-day hospitalization period, we may want to allocate (at least) half of the cost of the admission to the period prior to randomization and (at most) half to the period after randomization. Our parenthetical comments about "at least" and "at most" arise in part because of a general recognition that earlier days in the hospital are often more expensive than later days in the hospital.

If we are considering use of a repeated measures analysis of cost, we may have to make substantially more allocations. Also, as will be indicated in Chapter 6, a common approach to addressing censored data is to subdivide the period of follow-up into a number of partitions, for example, 1-month intervals, and to analyze the resulting estimates of monthly cost. Again, we would only want to use an administrative database that allows us to make such allocations.

Second, in cases where the administrative database includes payment information, the listed payments need not represent cost from the perspective adopted by the study. For example, in the U.S., if a database includes a measure of hospital charge, it is unlikely that there is any perspective for which this information would represent a good measure of cost, because in the U.S., charges for health care services do not reflect marginal opportunity cost [1], and very few payers actually pay charges. In these cases, we must identify a method for transforming the payment information into cost information. For example, in the U.S., a common method is to multiply charges times the cost-to-charge ratio.

Third, administrative data may not be updated continuously. Thus, if new postings of these data are made every 6 months or every 1 year, we may have to delay the analysis of a final dataset for a substantial length of time after the study has concluded follow-up.

Fourth, some sources of administrative data may not necessarily capture all medical service use and costs incurred by the participant. For example, in the U.S. VA database, many veterans may be dual users of both the VA system and U.S. Medicare or other insurance. For such patients medical services obtained from non-VA providers will not be available in the VA database.

Finally, Meenan [44] has reported that if participants are enrolled in different administrative databases, it may be difficult to pool data because of differences in systems of care, costing, and coding.

3.4. **Differential timing of expenditure**

When cost and effect are incurred at substantially different times, we must account for these differences in timing. The two main adjustments that must be considered are related to inflation for cost and time preference for cost and effect. Inflation refers to the general upward price movement of goods and services over time. Time preference, or discounting, refers to our differential valuation of a good or service, depending upon when the good or service is consumed. The two concepts are not the same: we would experience time preference even if there were no inflation.

The presence of inflation and time preference indicate that cost and effect in different time periods are not directly comparable. Comparison requires conversion to a common time period, for example the first year of the trial or the year the trial's results will be reported.

3.4.1. Inflation

If we use constant price weights to value all service use in the trial – for example 2006 Australian DRG payments – we need not adjust for inflation, even if medical service use is measured over a period of years. If, however, we use price weights from different time periods, for example 2006 price weights to value medical service use in 2006 and 2007 price weights to value medical service use in 2007, the cost of the medical service use in the two years can only be equated if we adjust for inflation. If we adopt the first year of the trial as the common time period in which all cost will be expressed, the usual formula for this adjustment is given by:

$$\sum_t \frac{C_t}{(1+i)^{(t-1)}}$$

where t equals time period (indexed from 1 to n); c_t equals cost in time t, and i equals the rate of inflation. We raise $(1 + i)$ to the $(t - 1)$ power, because in the first period, we do not adjust for inflation $((1 + i)^0 = 1)$; in the second period, we adjust for inflation for one period $((1 + i)^1 = 1 + i)$; etc. Alternatively, if cost is constant throughout the period, some have proposed use of the following formula:

$$\sum_t \frac{C_t}{(1+i)^{(t-0.5)}},$$

This formula is equivalent to adjusting for inflation as if cost were incurred at the middle of each interval.

3.4.2. Time preference

The formula used to account for time preference is similar to that used to account for inflation:

$$\sum_t \frac{C_t}{(1+r)^{(t-1)}},$$

where r equals the "real" discount rate. The real rate, which does not include an adjustment for inflation, can be contrasted with the nominal discount rate $\{[(1+r)(1+i)]^{(t-1)}\}$, which adjusts for both time preference and inflation. We use the convention of raising $(1+r)$ to the $(t-1)$ power so that discounting is consistent between a study in which follow-up lasts less than a year – for which common advice is to ignore discounting – and the first year of a study in which follow-up lasts for multiple years.

3.4.3. Sources for the inflation and discount rates

The most common source for deriving adjustment factors to account for inflation is the consumer price index. When adjusting the cost of medical service use, we often use the medical care component of the consumer price index (see Table 3.4). When adjusting cost in other sectors of the economy, we should consider using the cost component of the consumer price index that best represents the other services we are including in the estimate of cost. For simplicity, some authors use the overall consumer price index rather than the more specific sub-scales.

The theory used to derive the appropriate discount rate is substantially more complicated than that used to identify the appropriate inflation rate. For example, identification of an appropriate discount rate for a publicly provided health investment requires us to consider the source of the funds – are they coming from investment or from consumption? – as well as how the results of the investment will be used – will they go to investment or to consumption? [45]. Furthermore, we may consider modifying the discount rate we adopt to correct distortions in the economy that arise because of differences between the social rate of time preference and the rate of return on private investment.

Possibly as a means of avoiding this complexity, guidelines that consider the typical flows of resources have been proposed. Current practice in the U.S. and many other developed countries is to use a discount rate of 3% per year [46]. The discount rate may be higher in less developed countries, because their limited means may force them to focus more on meeting current needs at the expense of being sure they can meet more distant needs.

3.4.4. When to adjust for inflation and discounting

A number of common trial design features lead to the need to adjust for either inflation or time preference including the fact that trials may enroll participants during a very short period of time or their enrollment may stretch over several years. Follow-up of participants in trials may last for short periods of time, or it may stretch over several years. Finally, investigators may choose to value medical service use by use of constant price weights (e.g., use of the

Table 3.4 Consumer price index

Year	U.S.*			U.K.**		
	All items	Medical care	Medical care services	Pay and Health Service Cost Index	Pay Cost Index	Health Service Cost Index
1991	136.2	177.0	177.1	8.7	9.2	7.2
1992	140.3	190.1	190.5	10.1	11.5	6.5
1993	144.5	201.4	202.9	6.9	7.9	4.7
1994	148.2	211.0	213.4	3.4	4.2	1.4
1995	152.4	220.5	224.2	2.6	3.4	0.9
1996	156.9	228.2	232.4	4.0	4.4	3.2
1997	160.5	234.6	239.1	2.8	3.3	1.5
1998	163.0	242.1	246.8	1.7	2.5	0.4
1999	166.6	250.6	255.1	4.0	4.9	2.5
2000	172.2	260.8	266.0	4.5	6.9	1.2
2001	177.1	272.8	278.8	4.2	7.2	-0.3
2002	179.9	285.6	292.9	5.1	8.3	0.1
2003	184.0	297.1	306.0	3.6	5.0	1.3
2004	188.9	310.1	321.3	5.5	7.3	2.5

*http://data.bls.gov/cgi-bin/surveymost?cu. U.S. City Average, Not seasonally adjusted, base period: 1982–84 = 100.

**Hospital and Community Health Services (HCHS) pay and price inflation.

same price weight whether service use occurs in 2006 or 2010) or by use of time-varying price weights (e.g., by use of billing data from hospitals or physicians).

The decision about whether or not we must adjust for inflation relates to whether we choose to value medical service use by use of constant or time-varying price weights. The latter would occur, for example, if we used hospital billing data to cost out inpatient care observed in a multi-year trial. In other words, if overall trial follow-up lasts more than a year and if we use time-varying price weights, we will need to adjust for inflation.

The decision about whether or not we must adjust for time preference relates to the length of follow-up for individual participants in the trial. If per participant follow-up is longer than one year, we will have to adjust for time preference. If, on the other hand, per participant follow-up is less than a year and we use constant price weights to value medical service use, we need not account for either inflation or time preference. These relationships are summarized in Table 3.5.

The following examples may make these recommendations more concrete. Suppose a trial follows participants for 4 years and records inpatient service use within the case report form. At the end of follow-up, the investigators obtain a set of national price weights from one year (e.g., 2010) and use them to value service use observed in each of the four years of observation. In this case, we would not adjust for inflation, because we are using a constant set of price weights. We would, however, adjust for time preference, because individual participants' inpatient care occurred in more than one year.

Suppose that in a second trial participants are enrolled during a 3-year period, but each is followed for 1 year only. In addition, the investigators collect hospital bills to estimate inpatient cost. In this case, we would need to adjust for inflation, because hospital bills are coming from 3 different years, and inflation will make them noncomparable. We need not, however, account for time preference, because no participant's follow-up extends more than a year.

Table 3.5 Features of trial design and their effect on whether or not we should adjust for inflation and time preference

| Price weight | Per patient follow-up | |
	Less than 1 year	More than 1 year
Constant	Do not adjust for inflation; do not discount	Do not adjust for inflation; discount
Time varying	Adjust for inflation; do not discount	Adjust for inflation; discount

Suppose that in a third trial participants are enrolled during a 3-year period, that each is followed for 4 years, and that investigators collect hospital bills to estimate inpatient cost. In this case, we would need to account for both inflation and time preference.

Finally, suppose that in a fourth trial participants are enrolled during a 6-month period and each is followed for 6 months. The investigators either collect bills or obtain a single set of national price weights to value medical service use. In this case, we would neither adjust for inflation – because generally there would be little if any inflation in the observed cost estimates – nor adjust for time preference – because cost was incurred within a single year.

3.5. **Summary**

To recap, we commonly estimate the cost outcome of a trial by multiplying medical service use by a set or sets of price weights for these services. Two of the most common sources for price weights are national tariffs and center-specific price weights. National tariffs have a number of strengths, including that they represent what is spent by governments. Center-specific price weights, on the other hand, may give a more accurate estimate of the cost that was actually incurred in the trial. It is an open question if national tariffs are better than center-specific price weights for addressing national resource allocation questions if center-specific resource use is not representative of national resource use.

If for reasons of data collection cost we identify price weights for a selected set of services, it is incumbent that we develop a method for imputing price weights for the other services that were observed in the trial. One approach is to use readily available price weights, such as those from DRG or HRG payment systems, to develop a prediction model for available price weights. If for reasons of data collection cost we identify price weights for a selected set of centers or countries that participated in the trial, we should try to maximize the number of centers or countries in which price weights are collected rather than trying to maximize the number of price weights that are collected per center or country.

For a number of reasons, including potential biases that can arise due to substitution effects, we should multiply center-specific price weight estimates times center-specific quantities. For those centers and countries for which price weights are unavailable, price weights should be borrowed from similar centers and countries. Similarity can be defined along a number of dimensions, such as primary, secondary, or tertiary level of care or similarities in health care expenditures.

Finally, when cost and effect is incurred at substantially different times, we need to adjust for inflation and time preference. The actual adjustments that need to be made depend on the length of enrollment, the length of follow-up of participants, and the method one chooses to cost out medical service use.

References

1. Finkler SA. The distinction between costs and charges. *Ann Intern Med*. 1982; 96: 102–9.

2. Beck EJ, Beecham J, Mandalia S, Griffith R, Walters MDS, Boulton M, Miller DL. What is the cost of getting the price wrong? *J Public Health Med*. 1999; 21: 311–17.

3. Heerey A, McGowan B, Ryan M, Barry M. Microcosting versus DRGs in the provision of cost estimates for use in pharmacoeconomic evaluation. *Expert Rev Pharmacoeconomics Outcomes Res*. 2002; 2: 29–33.

4. Shwartz M, Young DW, Siegrist R. The ratio of costs to charges: how good a basis for estimating costs? *Inquiry* 1995; 32: 476–81.

5. Rittenhouse BE, Dulissec B, Stinnett AA. At what price significance? The effect of price estimates on statistical inference in economic evaluation. *Health Econ*. 1999; 8: 213–19.

6. Reed SD, Friedman JY, Gnanasakthy A, Schulman KA. Comparison of hospital costing methods in an economic evaluation of a multinational clinical trial. *Int J Technol Assess Health Care* 2003; 19: 395–406.

7. Chumney ECG, Biddle AK, Simpson KN, Weinberger M, Magruder KM, Zelman WN. The effect of cost construction based on either DRG or ICD-9 codes or risk group stratification on the resulting cost-effectiveness ratios. *Pharmacoeconomics* 2004; 22: 1209–16.

8. Taira DA, Seto TB, Siegrist R, Cosgrove R, Berezin R, Cohen DJ. Comparison of analytic approaches for the economic evaluation of new technologies alongside multicenter clinical trials. *Am Heart J*. 2003; 145: 452–8.

9. Goeree R, Gafni A, Hannah M, Myhr T, Blackhouse G. Hospital selection for unit cost estimates in multicentre economic evaluations. Does the choice of hospitals make a difference? *Pharmacoeconomics* 1999; 15: 561–72.

10. Schulman K, Burke J, Drummond M, Davies L, Carlsson P, Gruger J, Harris A, Lucioni C, Gisbert R, Llana T, Tom E, Bloom B, Willke R, Glick H. Resource costing for multinational neurologic clinical trials: methods and results. *Health Econ*. 1998; 7: 629–38.

11. Glick HA, Orzol SM, Tooley JF, Polsky D, Mauskopf JO. Design and analysis of unit cost estimation studies: how many hospital diagnoses? how many countries? *Health Econ*. 2003; 12: 517–27.

12. Adam T, Evans DB, Murray, CJL. *Econometric estimation of country-specific hospital costs*. http://www.resource-allocation.com/content/1/1/3

13. British Medical Association and Royal Pharmaceutical Society of Great Britain. British National Formulary 39. London: British Medical Association, 2000.

14. Pauly MV. Measures of costs and benefits for drugs in cost effectiveness analysis. Chapter 10. In *Promoting and Coping with Pharmaceutical Innovation: An International*

Perspective, edited by F. Sloan and C.R. Hsieh. Cambridge: Cambridge University Press, In press.

15. Riteco JA, de Heij LJM, van Luijn JCF, Wolff I. *Dutch Guidelines for Pharmacoeconomic Research*. Amstelveen: College Voor Zorgverzekeringen, 1999.

16. Oostenbrink JB, Koopmanschap MA, Rutten FFH. Standardisation of costs. The Dutch manual for costing in economic evaluations. *Pharmacoeconomics* 2002; 20: 443–54.

17. Garattini L, Giuliani G, Pagano E. A model for calculating costs of hospital wards: an Italian experience. *J Manage Med*. 1999; 13: 71–82.

18. Oostenbrink JB, Buijs-Van der Woude T, van Agthoven M, Koopmanschap MA, Rutten FF. Unit costs of inpatient hospital days. *Pharmacoeconomics* 2003; 21: 263–71.

19. Scullen C, Scott MG, Gribbin M, McElnay JC. A HRG-based costing model for estimating pharmacy costs associated with surgical procedures. *J Clin Pharm Ther*. 2004; 29: 257–62.

20. Bridges M, Jacobs P. Obtaining estimates of marginal cost by DRG. *Healthc Financ Manage*. 1986; 10: 40–6.

21. Dean J, Edbrook D, Corcoran M. The critical care national cost block programme: implementing a standard costing method on a national scale. *Care of the Critically Ill* 2002: 18.

22. Negrini D, Kettle A, Sheppard L, Mills GH, Edbrooke DL. The cost of a hospital ward in Europe. *J Health Organ Manage*. 2004; 18: 195–205.

23. Granneman TW, Brown RS, Pauly MV. Estimating hospital costs. A multiple-output analysis. *J Health Econ*. 1986; 5: 107–27.

24. Gaynor M, Anderson GF. Uncertain demand, the structure of hospital costs, and the cost of empty hospital beds. *J Health Econ*. 1995; 14: 291–317.

25. Li T, Rosenman R. Estimating hospital costs with a generalized Leontief function. *Health Econ*. 201; 10: 523–38.

26. Finkler SA. Cost finding for high-technology, high-cost services: current practice and a possible alternative. *Health Care Manage Rev*. 1980; 5: 17–29.

27. Kirk R. Using workload analysis and acuity systems to facilitate quality and productivity. *J Nurs Adm*. 1990; 20: 21–30.

28. Oddone E, Weinberger M, Hurder A, Henderson W, Simel D. Measuring activities in clinical trials using random work sampling: implications for cost-effectiveness analysis and measurement of the intervention. *J Clin Epi*. 1995; 48: 1011–8.

29. Pelletier D, Duffield C. Work sampling: valuable methodology to define nursing practice patterns. *Nurs Health Sci*. 2003; 5: 31–8.

30. Glick HA, Kinosian B, McBride L, Williford WO, Bauer MS. Clinical nurse specialist care managers' time commitments in a disease-management program for bipolar disorder. *Bipolar Disord*. 2004; 6: 452–9.

31. Iglar AM, Osland CS, Ploetz PA, Thielke TS. Time and cost requirements for decentralized pharmacist activities. *Am J Hosp Pharm*. 1990; 47: 572–8.

32. Harpole LH, Stechuchak KM, Saur CD, Steffens DC, Unutzer J, Eugene Oddone E. Implementing a disease management intervention for depression in primary care: a random work sampling study. *Gen Hosp Psychiatry* 2003; 25; 238–45.

33. Organization for Economic Cooperation and Development. *Main Economic Indicators*, Paris March 2006.

34. Bleaney M. Does long run purchasing power-parity hold within the European monetary system? *J Econ Stud.* 1992; 19: 66–72.

35. Raikou M, Briggs A, Gray A, Mcguire A. Centre-specific or average unit costs in multi-centre studies? Some theory and simulation. *Health Econ.* 2000; 9: 191–8.

36. Office of Economic Cooperation and Development. *OECD Health Data 2005.* Paris, France: OECD Electronic Publications, 2006.

37. French MT, Dunlop LJ, Zarkin GA, McGeary KA, McLellan AT. A structured instrument for estimating the economic cost of drug abuse treatment. The Drug Abuse Treatment Cost Analysis Program (DATCAP). *J Subst Abuse Treat.* 1997; 14: 445–55.

38. French MT, Roebuck MC, McLellan AT. Cost estimation when time and resources are limited: the brief DATCAP. *J Subst Abuse Treat.* 2004; 27: 187–93.

39. Anderson DW, Bowland BJ, Cartwright WS, Bassin G. Service-level costing of drug abuse treatment. *J Subst Abuse Treat.* 1998; 15: 201–11.

40. Barrett B, Byford S, Seivewright H, Coopers S, Tyrer P. Service costs for severe personality disorder at a special hospital. *Crim Behav Ment Health* 2005; 15: 184–90.

41. The Diabetes Prevention Program Research Group. Costs associated with the primary prevention of type 2 diabetes mellitus in the Diabetes Prevention Program. *Diabetes Care* 2003; 26: 36–47.

42. Starkey R, Moore L, Campbell R, Sidaway M, Bloor M and ASSIST (A Stop Smoking In Schools Trial). Rationale, design and conduct of a comprehensive evaluation of a school-based peer-led anti-smoking intervention in the UK: the ASSIST cluster randomised trial [ISRCTN55572965]. *BMC Public Health* 2005; 5: 43–52.

43. Ronckers ET, Groot W, Steenbakkers M, Ruland E, Ament A. Costs of the "Hartslag Limburg" community heart health intervention. *BMC Public Health* 2006; 6: 51–60.

44. Meenan RT, Goodman MJ, Fishman PA, Hornbrook MC, O'Keeffe-Rosetti MC, Bachman DJ. Issues in pooling administrative data for economic evaluation. *Am J Manag Care* 2002; 8: 45–53.

45. Lind RC. A primer on the major issues relating to the discount rate for evaluating national energy options. In *Discounting for Time and Risk in Energy Policy*. Baltimore: Johns Hopkins University Press, 1982, pp. 21–94.

46. Gold MR, Siegel JE, Russel LB, Weinstein MC (editors). *Cost-Effectiveness in Health and Medicine.* Oxford: Oxford University Press, 1996.

Chapter 4

Assessing quality-adjusted life years

Economic evaluation requires the measurement of both cost and effect. There are no limits to the types of measures of effect that we can include in a cost-effectiveness ratio. For example, they can range from changes in biological markers such as blood pressure, cholesterol, or glucose, to intermediate health outcomes such as cases of illness avoided, number of successful treatments, or to more final outcomes such as lives saved or years of life gained.

For our results to aid in decision making, however, we need to adopt a measure of effectiveness (1) that allows direct comparison of therapies across a number of domains, (2) that allows comparison across therapeutic areas and illnesses, and (3) for which we generally understand how much we are willing to pay for a unit of effect. As we indicated in Chapter 2, while there is no full agreement surrounding willingness to pay for a quality-adjusted life year (QALY), there are commonly accepted ranges for these values. Thus, for this reason, and because the ratio of cost per QALY saved is the recommended outcome for cost-effectiveness analysis [1], in this chapter, we focus on issues of measurement of QALYs in trials.

A second means of overcoming the problem of understanding how much we are willing to pay for a unit of effect is to directly assess willingness to pay, in other words, to perform cost-benefit analysis. While we do not discuss this method, there has been a growing literature about the assessment of willingness to pay for health and health care, so much so that willingness to pay studies are appearing in specialty medical journals [2–6]. Three reviews that interested readers may find helpful include those by Diener *et al.* [7], Klose [8], and Olsen and Smith [9].

In the following sections, we introduce QALYs, describe and compare three prescored preference assessment instruments; describe and compare three direct elicitation methods for assessing preferences; discuss construction of the QALY outcome and frequency of administration of preference assessment instruments, and discuss the role of responsiveness in the choice of these instruments.

4.1. **Quality-adjusted life years (QALYs)**

QALYs are an economic outcome that combines preferences for both length of survival and its quality into a single measure. QALY or preference scores generally range between 0 (death) and 1 (perfect health). For example, a health state with a preference score of 0.8 indicates that a year in that state is worth 0.8 of a year with perfect health, although there can be states worse than death with preference scores less than 0.

Methods for the assessment of QALYs are often differentiated by whether or not they incorporate preference for risk, which technically yields a utility when they do and a value when they do not. For example, this characteristic is one of the differentiating features of the three direct preference elicitation methods that we describe below. In the following discussion, we will refer to preference assessment, preference scores, or preferences when we are referring to generic assessment of QALYs. We will reserve the terms utility assessment, utility scores, or utilities and value assessment, values scores, and values for our references to methods that are used to derive utilities or values, respectively.

Another differentiating characteristic of methods for the assessment of QALYs is whether they are measured as a series of valuations of current health – usually by use of prescored instruments or direct elicitation methods – or whether they are measured by use of an explicit preference mapping for years of survival and their quality. One such mapping, which was reported in the classic study by McNeil *et al.* [10], is shown in Fig. 4.1. Because most preference assessment in clinical trials is based on a series of valuations of current health, in the following discussion, we address methods for this assessment and do not discuss how one develops a preference mapping.

In the pragmatic world of economic evaluation in trials, we often ignore these distinctions between utilities and values and between preference measures that reflect different durations of symptomatology versus those that value current health. But they do have implications. One of these is that, as with our discussion of price weights in Chapter 3, most of our methods yield second-best approximations of what we actually would like to measure.

A third differentiating characteristic relates to whose preferences we are measuring. The Panel on Cost Effectiveness in Health and Medicine [1] has recommended a reference case analysis that uses community preferences to value health (Chapter 4, Recommendation 4, p. 122) as well as a sensitivity analysis that uses preferences of persons with the condition (Chapter 4, Recommendation 5, p. 122).

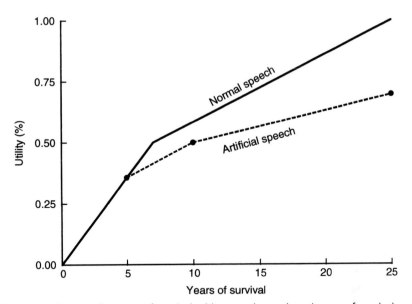

Fig. 4.1 Preferences for years of survival with normal speech and years of survival with artificial speech. The normal speech curve was derived by use of standard gambles; the artificial speech curve was derive by use of time trade-offs. Source: McNeil *et al.* [10].

From McNeil BJ, Weichselbaum, Pauker SG. Speech and Survival Trade offs between quality and quantity of life in laryngeal Cancer. *NEJM* 1981; 305: 982-8 (c)1981 Massachusetts Medical Society. All rights reserved.

Turning back to the pragmatic, there are a number of methods that are commonly used for the measurement of QALYs as a series of valuations of current health. They all yield what we refer to as preference scores which are integrated over time to yield a measure of QALYs (see Section 4.4).

One of the two dominant approaches for QALY measurement uses prescored health state classification instruments, and is sometimes referred to as indirect utility assessment. These instruments have trial participants report their functional status across a variety of domains. Preference scores are then derived from scoring rules that have usually been developed by use of samples from the general public. These instruments are considered to satisfy the "community preferences" recommendation of the Panel on Cost Effectiveness. Rasanen *et al.* [11] reported in 2006 that prescored instruments were used in 76% of studies that measured QALYs among patients.

The second dominant approach for estimating preference scores directly elicits participants' preferences for their current health. When administered to study participants, these methods yield measures of patient preference.

A third approach that is less used in trial-based analysis describes disease scenarios to members of the general public and directly elicits their preferences for these scenarios. Participants in the trial are then categorized into the different scenarios and their QALYs estimated. We do not discuss this method below. Rather, in what follows, we describe prescored instruments and direct elicitation methods.

4.2. Prescored instruments

One common approach for assessing QALYs in trials is to use a prescored instrument. A number of these instruments are currently available for the measurement of preference scores for current health. Examples include the EuroQol instrument [12,13], the Health Utilities Index Mark 2 (HUI2) or Mark 3 (HUI3) [14,15], the SF-6D [16], the Quality of Well-Being Scale (QWB) [17], the 15D [18], and the Disability and Distress Index [19,20].

Most of these instruments ask participants or their proxies to report on the health status of the patient. For example, the HUI2 has patients record their level of functioning for seven domains. They then use predetermined weights to compute preference scores. With at least one instrument (i.e., the EuroQol), patients also rate their current health.

The EuroQol instrument, the HUI2, and the HUI3 are three of the most commonly used prescored preference assessment instruments. In fact, Rasanen et al. [11] have reported that the EuroQol instrument is the most used of any instrument, prescored or directly elicited. All these three instruments share features of ease of use – for example high completion rates and the ability to be filled out in 5 min or less – and they all have been used to assess preferences for a wide variety of diseases. We describe these instruments below.

4.2.1. The EuroQol instrument

The EuroQol instrument is made up of two parts, a health state classification instrument (EQ-5D) and its attendant scoring rule – which yields a preference score that represents the general public's preference for the health state – and a 100-point visual analog scale – which yields a measure of patient preference. We describe the latter part of this instrument in Section 4.3.

The EQ-5D health state classification instrument has five domains, mobility, self-care, usual activities, pain/discomfort, and anxiety/depression. Each domain is defined by three levels of function from good to poor, which are generally worded, "I have no problems..."; "I have some problems..."; and "I am unable....." The three levels for each of the five domains can be used to define 243 (3^5) health states.

The principal scoring rule was developed by Dolan [21] by use of time trade-off responses from a representative sample of 2997 noninstitutionalized adults from England, Scotland, and Wales. Other scoring rules have been proposed, for example those by Johnson *et al.* [22] and by Polsky *et al.* [23], but they generally have not been used in the literature.

4.2.2. **HUI2**

The HUI2 has seven domains with varying numbers of levels depending on the domain. The domains and number of levels include sensory with four levels, mobility with five, emotion with five, cognition with four, self-care with four, pain with five, and fertility with three. A number of investigators have omitted the fertility domain when they have not believed that it is affected by the disease in question [24]. The multiple levels of the seven domains can be used to define 24,000 health states.

The index has two multiplicative scoring rules that were derived from responses of 293 parents of school children drawn from the general population in Canada (because the rules were initially developed to evaluate a therapy for childhood cancer) [14]. We focus on the utility scoring rule that was developed by use of standard gambles, but there is also a value scoring rule that was developed by use of a visual analog scale. At least one other scoring rule has been proposed [25].

4.2.3. **HUI3**

The HUI3 has eight domains each with five or six levels depending on the domain. The domains and number of levels include vision with six levels, hearing with six, speech with five, ambulation with six, dexterity with six, emotion with five, cognition with six and pain with five. The levels of the domains can be used to define 972,000 health states.

As with the HUI2, the HUI3 has two multiplicative scoring rules. For the HUI3, they were derived from responses from a random sample of 256 adults drawn from the general population in Hamilton, Ontario [15]. Also, as with the HUI2, we focus on the utility scoring rule that was developed by use of standard gambles, but there is also a value scoring rule that was developed by use of a visual analog scale.

4.2.4. **Comparison of instruments**

Table 4.1 describes several similarities and differences between the three instruments. The Dolan scoring rule for the EQ-5D yields only 1 health state with a preference score between 0.9 and 1 (the state representing full function with a preference score of 1.0); the utility scoring rule for the HUI2 yields 27 health states with preference scores between 0.9 and 1; and the utility scoring rule for the HUI3 yields 14 such states.

The EQ-5D has 84 states worse than death, and its lowest possible score is −0.594. The HUI2 has 63 states worse than death, and its lowest score is −0.025. The HUI3, on the other hand, has 642,884 states worse than death, and its lowest score is −0.359.

Table 4.1 Comparison of distribution of states for the three instruments

	EQ-5D	HUI2*	HUI3
States with scores ≥ 0.9 (N)	1	27	14
States with scores < 0.0 (N)	84	63	642,884
Average score (equal weighting)	0.137	0.286	−0.101
Lowest score	−0.594	−0.025	−0.359

*Derived by use of the "utility" scoring rule based on standard gambles.

Finally, the average score for the 243 states of the EQ-5D is 0.137, in part because 35% of states are worse than death. The average score for the 24,000 states of the HUI2 is 0.286. Lastly, the average score for the 972,000 states of the HUI3 is −0.101, again principally because 66% of states are worse than death. In sum, these features suggest that the instruments focus on different ranges of the QALY spectrum.

A number of authors have compared two or three of these instruments in the same patient population. As shown in Table 4.2, with the exception of the large study by Luo *et al.* [31] there is substantial evidence that the HUI2 yields significantly higher scores than either the EQ-5D or the HUI3. Evidence about the EQ-5D and HUI3 is less consistent. One large study by McDonough *et al.* [33] found that the EQ-5D scores were significantly lower than HUI3 scores; another large study by Luo *et al.* [31] found that the EQ-5D scores were significantly higher than the HUI3 scores. These differences may have to do with the severity of the patients whose preferences were elicited in the two studies. In most of the other studies, there were no significant differences between the EQ-5D and the HUI3.

Conner-Spady and Suarez-Almazor's study [29] is one of the few that has compared changes in preference scores yielded by the EQ-5D and HUI3. They found that among patients who improved clinically, the preference scores from the EQ-5D had a significantly larger mean improvement than did the preference scores from the HUI3; among patients who worsened clinically, the preference scores from the EQ-5D had a significantly larger mean decrement than those from the HUI3. Blanchard *et al.'s* [26] study is one of the few to evaluate the relative responsiveness of the HUI2 and HUI3. They found that the change in HUI3 preferences scores was significantly larger than the change in HUI2 scores.

Most of these studies that evaluated correlations between the preference scores found them to be correlated; most that evaluated correlations between

Table 4.2 Comparison of preference scores derived by use of the EQ-5D, HUI2, and HUI3

Study	N	EQ-5D	HUI2	HUI3	Notes*
Blanchard *et al.* [26]					
Presurgery	90	–	0.60 (0.17)	0.47 (0.21)	(A)
Postsurgery	90	–	0.77 (0.27)	0.72 (0.18)	(B)
Bosch and Hunink [27]					
0 months	88	0.57 (0.25)	–	0.66 (0.20)	(A)
1 month	84	0.79 (0.23)	–	0.77 (0.21)	(B)
3 months	84	0.77 (0.26)	–	0.78 (0.22)	(B)
12 months	72	0.75 (0.21)	–	0.77 (0.22)	(B)
Chong *et al.* [28]					
No biopsy	35	0.69 (0.35)	–	0.73 (0.32)	(B)
Mild/moderate	44	0.73 (0.32)	–	0.76 (0.25)	(B)
Compensated cirrhosis	24	0.74 (0.21)	–	0.74 (0.21)	(B)
Transplant	30	0.70 (0.20)	–	0.69 (0.21)	(B)
Sustained virological response	36	0.77 (0.26)	–	0.83 (0.20)	(B)
Conner-Spady and Suarez-Almazor [29]	161	0.49 (0.31)	–	0.50 (0.27)	(B)
Feeny *et al.* [30]	264	–	0.92 (0.13)	0.84 (0.19)	(A)
Luo [31] *et al.*†	4048	0.87 (0.01)	0.86 (0.01)	0.81 (0.01)	(C)
Marra *et al.* [32]	302	0.66 (0.24)	0.71 (0.20)	0.53 (0.29)	(D)
McDonough *et al.* [33]	2097	0.39 (0.33)	0.59 (0.22)	0.45 (0.27)	(D)
Neumann *et al.* [34]‡	679	–	0.53 (0.21)	0.22 (0.26)	(A)
Siderowf *et al.* [35]	97	0.59 (0.27)	0.93 (0.17)	–	(A)
Suarez-Almazor *et al.* [36]	46	0.38 (0.33)	0.49 (0.19)	–	

*Statistical tests based on means, SDs, and Ns reported in studies, and do not account for the fact that the same patients responded to all three instruments.

†Mean (SE).

‡Caregivers of patients.

(A) $p < 0.05$.

(B) No significant difference.

(C) HUI3 significantly lower than HUI2 and EQ-5D.

(D) All 3 pair-wise comparisons are significantly different.

the preference scores and convergent validity criteria found them to be correlated (data not shown). Most of the studies that evaluated responsiveness concluded that all of the instruments were responsive. Finally, most concluded that there was little evidence that one instrument was superior to another.

At the same time, there were isolated reports of less favorable findings for a specific instrument, most often the EQ-5D. For example, Luo *et al.* [31] noted that the EQ-5D demonstrated more ceiling effects than either the HUI2 or HUI3. Marra *et al.* [37] found that the test–retest reliability was acceptable for the HUI2 and HUI3, but was not acceptable for the EQ-5D (although they noted that (1) a previous study had shown the EQ-5D to be reliable in a similar patient population and (2) their retest interval of 5 weeks may have been long enough for patients' status to have changed). Finally, Suarez-Almazor *et al.* [36] reported that compared to the HUI2, the EQ-5D did not respond well at 3 months, but did at 6 months. But to recap, the sense of the literature is that none of the instruments performs better than the other.

4.2.5. Choice between instruments

A number of authors have concluded that while all three instruments appear to be measuring the quality of life, the constructs they are measuring are not identical and the preference scores, and thus QALYs derived from them, differ [29,33,36,38]. As Conner-Spady and Suarez-Almazor [29] note, the instruments' "index scores are not interchangeable in the calculation of longitudinal-based QALYs" (p. 799).

Given that all three instruments are meant to be measuring the same construct – QALYs, which should be comparable across diseases and patients – and given that there is little evidence that supports the superiority of one instrument over another, the fact that the instruments disagree is problematic. While a number of authors have provided advice about choosing among the instruments, it has been very general in nature. For example, Conner-Spady and Suarez-Almazor [29] have recommended that choice should be guided by whether the instrument is appropriate for its intended use. Unfortunately, for many diseases, investigators have found reasonable correlations between the three instruments' scores and reasonable correlations between these scores and independent convergent validity criteria. These findings suggest that all the three instruments are generally appropriate for their intended use.

Alternately, McDonough *et al.* [33] have recommended that "practical and design aspects of measurement tools may indicate which tool would be better suited for measurement of the quality of life" (p. 1328). However, except for differences in the timeframes used by the instruments, the authors did not identify which practical or design aspects might make one instrument more suitable than another.

One might suppose that the absence of a domain that would be expected to be related to disease might justify adoption of one instrument compared with another. For example, the absence of a domain related to cognition might suggest that the EQ-5D would not be as useful among patients with Alzheimer's disease as would the HUI2, which has such a domain. Our unpublished data, on the other hand, do not reveal dramatic differences in the associations between EQ-5D and HUI2 scores and a number of convergent validity criteria. One reason may be that for the EQ-5D problems with cognition are reflected as problems with usual activities.

On our reading of the literature, for most diseases, it does not seem as though the widespread direct comparison of the instruments is providing an answer about which instrument should be used in which circumstances. As Siderowf *et al.* [35] have noted, part of the problem is due to the fact that while correlation between the instruments' scores and convergent validity criteria is important, health preference is not the same as health status. Thus, if one instrument has higher correlations with convergent validity criteria, or if one instrument is more responsive than another, that does not necessarily translate into it being a better instrument. However, before throwing up our hands and suggesting you draw straws, we will reconsider this issue after we review how the results of the prescored instruments compare with the results of direct elicitation of preferences from study participants.

4.3. **Direct elicitation from participants**

A second common approach for assessing QALYs in trials is to directly elicit preferences from study participants. The three most common methods for doing so are the standard gamble, the time trade-off, and the rating scale. Rasanen *et al.* [11] have reported that among studies that have directly elicited preferences from patients as part of an economic evaluation, the standard gamble has been used 21% of the time, the time trade-off has been used 42% of the time, and the rating scale 37%. These numbers vary slightly from those previously reported by Morimoto and Fukui [39].

We briefly describe each of these methods in turn below.

4.3.1. **Standard gamble**

A standard gamble asks participants to trade-off a certain, intermediate, outcome for a gamble for a better and worse outcome. For example, the participant might be asked to choose between living with current health for 10 years versus a $p/1-p$ gamble of living with full function for 10 years or dying immediately. Standard gambles satisfy the axioms of expected utility theory as proposed by von Neumann and Morgenstern [40]. This theory states that when making decisions based on maximization of expected utility, the measures of outcome should reflect preference measured with risk. As Drummond *et al.* [41]

have noted, in addition to being risk based, standard gambles – unlike rating scales – also require that participants choose between health outcomes.

While there are a number of methods available for framing a standard gamble, the most common one used for direct elicitation of preference for current health is to pose what is referred to as a probability-equivalent standard gamble. The example above represents such a gamble. As in the example, one approach for presenting a probability-equivalent gamble is to describe a level of health for a specific length of survival, for example 10 years or the number of years that represent the participant's life expectancy. Alternately, some authors omit the description of the length of survival and offer current health with length of survival unspecified versus a gamble for best and worst imaginable health (see discussion below about the impact of time horizon on responses to the gamble). In either case, the participant is asked to identify p such that she is indifferent between the certain outcome and the gamble.

We interpret the probability that makes the respondent indifferent between the two choices as the preference or utility score. We do so because by indicating indifference, the respondent states that the utility of the certain outcome is identical to the utility of the gamble. Under expected utility theory, the utility of the gamble is made up of p times the utility of the best outcome, for example full functioning, which we assume has a utility of 1.0, plus $1-p$ times the utility of the worst outcome, which drops out of the equation because we assume its utility equals 0. The gamble is illustrated in Fig. 4.2.

4.3.2. Time trade-off

A time trade-off asks participants to trade-off morbid years for healthy years [42]. A participant is asked to choose between living some length of

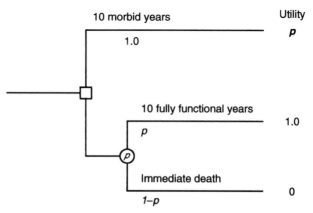

Fig. 4.2 Probability equivalent standard gamble.

time – for example, 10 years or the number of years that represent the participant's life expectancy – with her current health versus living a shorter period of time with fully functional health. The participant is asked to identify the number of years with fully functional health that makes her indifferent between the longer morbid life expectancy and the shorter fully-functional life expectancy.

Unlike standard gambles, time trade-offs do not satisfy the axioms of expected utility theory, because they are not measured with risk. Like standard gambles, on the other hand, they do require that participants choose between health outcomes.

To obtain a preference score, we divide the number of healthy years identified by the participant by the number of morbid years. For example, if the participant reported that she was indifferent between 7 healthy years and 10 morbid years, the resulting preference score would be 0.7.

4.3.3. Rating scale

A rating scale – also referred to as visual analog scale or feeling thermometer – asks participants to rate how good or bad their current health is on a 0–1 or 0–100 scale. Zero often represents worst imaginable health or death; 1 often represents "best imaginable health" or "full health" (see Fig. 4.3). The EuroQol 100-point visual analog scale [12] is a commonly used visual analog scale. It is drawn as a 20 cm vertical line with its lower end representing the worst imaginable health state (0) and its upper end representing the best imaginable health state (100). It is subdivided into 10 unit intervals with subinterval tic marks (http://gs1.q4matics.com/EuroqolPublishWeb/#). More generally, as Green et al. [43] have noted, rating scales can vary in presentation in terms of length of the line, whether they are drawn vertically or horizontally, and whether or not they have intervals marked out with numbers. Some have argued that having intervals marked out with numbers can induce memory effects and clustering [44].

Rating scales neither satisfy the axioms of expected utility theory, nor do they require that participants choose between health outcomes.

If a rating scale ranges between 0 and 1, the point on the line selected by the participant represents her preference score; if the scale ranges between 0 and 100, the point on the line divided by 100 represents this score.

4.3.4. Search procedures and time horizons for standard gambles and time trade-offs

It is possible to administer standard gambles and time trade-offs by use of a single open-ended question, such as "Which p makes you indifferent?" or

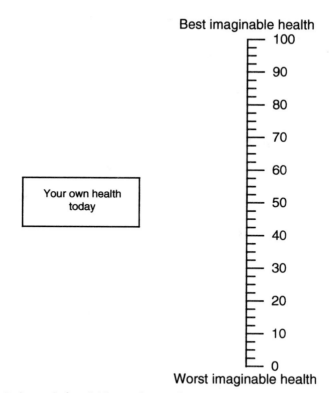

Fig. 4.3 Rating scale for eliciting preference for current health.

"How many years with full function make you indifferent?" However, they are more commonly administered by use of a series of close-ended questions. Using the standard gamble as an example, "Would you rather live with your current health for 10 years or would you choose a gamble in which you have a 90% chance of living 10 fully functional years and a 10% chance of dying immediately." The probabilities are changed and the question repeated until the respondent reports she is indifferent between the options.

When offered as a series of close-ended questions, the questions can ping-pong from high to low to high; they can offer probabilities or years of healthy survival in steps from the maximum to the minimum, referred to as titration down; they can offer them from the minimum to the maximum, referred to as titration up; or they can be posed by use of interval division search strategies [45,46], which are also referred to as bisecting search routines [47]. Lenert *et al.* [45] have reported that different search procedures can have strong and persistent effects on reported preference scores for both standard gambles and time trade-offs. This finding supports findings of an earlier study by Percy and Llewellyn-Thomas [48]. Hammerschmidt et al. [46], on the other hand, did not see significant differences between the results of mailed questionnaire standard gambles that used top-down versus bottom-up search procedures, which supports earlier findings by Tsevat et al. [49].

There is more consistency in the literature on the effect of time horizon on preferences assessed by use of standard gambles and time trade-offs. As Torrance et al. [42] noted in 1972, the preferences for highly confining health states appear to be a decreasing function of time, whereas preferences for inconvenient health states appear to be an increasing function of time. Most investigators who have empirically assessed the effect of time horizon have found that the longer the time horizon, the smaller the resulting preference scores. This finding holds for standard gambles [50,51], time trade-offs [10,52], and rating scales [51]. Bala et al. [53] suggest that their study also supports a finding that time horizon matters, in that 85% of patients had substantially different standard gamble responses depending on whether the time horizon of the gamble was 1 year or 20 years. However, given that the mean valuations for these two time horizons were within 0.01 of each other, it is not clear that their findings support the claim that mean QALYs differ by time horizon of elicitation.

An example of the magnitude of the impact of the use of differing time horizons is provided by McNeil et al. [10]. Table 4.3 shows three of the time trade-offs that were depicted in Fig. 4.1. When offered 25 morbid years, respondents reported a time trade-off of 12.5 healthy years (preference score = 0.5), whereas when offered 5 morbid years, they were unwilling to trade-off any year to be healthy (preference score of 1.0).

As a technical note, this lack of independence between preference scores and timeframes represents a violation of both the constant proportional risk attitude to survival duration assumption for standard gambles and the constant proportional time trade-off assumption for time trade-offs [54]. This violation

Table 4.3 QALY weights for impaired speech as measured by use of a time trade-off by McNeil et al. [10]

Morbid years	Healthy years	Preference score*
25	12.5	0.5
10	7	0.7
5	5	1.0

*Preference score = healthy years/morbid years.

has implications for the theoretical underpinnings of these methods. Again, technically speaking, as Loomes and McKenzie [54] have noted, it means that utility cannot be calculated "as expected length of life multiplied by a factor measuring the utility of survival duration in a particular health state relative to the utility of survival in excellent health." (p. 300).

Theory aside, what time horizons have investigators used in the literature? In reviewing 27 studies that asked patients (or in two cases, parents of patients) to rate their current health by use of the standard gamble, time trade-off, and rating scale, we found that seven used time horizons of 10 years or less, seven used horizons of 20–30 years, and 12 used life expectancy as the time horizon (i.e., time horizons tailored to each participant based on her age). It is unclear how much variability of results in the literature arises because of the use of these different time horizons.

4.3.5. Methods of administration

Standard gambles and time trade-offs are most commonly administered by use of an interview, often with the aid of chance boards, decision wheels, and pie charts; rating scales are usually self-administered as part of an interview. All three methods can be self-completed by participants [55,56]. There are a number of computer-directed questionnaires that can be used for their administration, including U-Titer [57], U-Maker [58], and iMPACT [59,60]. The Functional Limitation and Independence Rating (FLAIR) has been developed to support preference assessment in older, computer-inexperienced participants [61]. Investigators have also designed internet-based surveys of preference for specific studies [47,53].

van Wijck et al. [62] have reported that telephone interviews (preceded by a mailed survey) yield standard gamble and time trade-off results that are similar to those obtained by face-to-face interview. There is good evidence of the feasibility of use of rating scales in mailed, self-completed surveys [63,64]. Evidence for the feasibility of mailed, self-completed standard gambles appears more mixed. Ross et al. [65] and Littenberg et al. [66] have reported that a one-page paper standard gamble is a reliable measure of patient preference and is suitable for use in mailed surveys. Hammerschmidt et al. [46], on the other hand, have reported substantial feasibility problems for mailed, self-completed standard gambles.

Green et al. [43] provide a good summary of the practicality and reliability of the three methods. They report that there is substantial evidence supporting their practicality in terms of completion and response rates, and they discount claims that standard gambles are too complex or not intuitively obvious to participants. At the same time, they note that rating scales may be "slightly better in terms of response rate and cost." They also note that it appears as though the standard gamble and time trade-off methods "result in a larger number of refusals, missing values, and inconsistent responses" than do rating scales [43, p. 157]. Woloshin *et al.* [67] have more recently raised concerns about the quality of the results from standard gambles and time trade-offs among less numerate participants. Finally, Green *et al.* [43] report that all the three methods have acceptable levels of reliability, although they found some evidence that the time trade-off may have slightly better test–retest performance.

4.3.6. **Theoretical differences between the measures**

It is routinely pointed out that standard gambles are consistent with expected utility theory, and thus are theoretically superior to time trade-offs and rating scales (this claim seems to ignore the implications of the violation of the constant proportional risk attitude assumption). As Green *et al.* [43] indicate, some authors have argued that the fact that the time trade-off has participants make choices between health outcomes indicates that it is superior to the rating scale. While Green *et al.* do not appear to accept this argument, when linked with the claim that standard gambles and time trade-offs in practice yield similar results, there is a general gestalt in the literature that standard gambles and time trade-offs are relatively interchangeable, and that rating scales are an inferior method for the measurement of preference.

We do not want to take a position on this theoretical debate. We will point out that in the face of negative comments about the theoretical foundations of rating scales [68,69], Parkin and Devlin [70] have made a spirited defense of rating scale methods for use in economic evaluation. We instead turn to the empirical evidence comparing the results of the three elicitation procedures.

4.3.7. **Summary of findings from the three methods**

Table 4.4 summarizes the results from 27 studies that asked patients to rate their health by use of the standard gamble, time trade-off, and rating scale (references available from authors). The 27 studies reported results for 46 samples of participants, for example those with mild disease versus those with severe disease or the same patients prior to and after receiving of therapy. These studies included 4962 responses from all of the three methods. Comparison of the overall means across the studies confirms the suggestion in the literature that the difference between mean standard gamble and time trade-off responses (approximately 0.03) is much smaller than the difference between the mean standard gamble and rating scale responses (approximately 0.14). This finding is independent of whether we take the weighted average of the results from the 46 samples or we simply average the sample means.

Table 4.4 Comparison of preference scores derived by use of three direct elicitation methods

	N	Standard gamble	Time trade-off	Rating scale
Weighted average	4962	0.872	0.844	0.741
Unweighted average	46	0.857	0.825	0.707
		SG versus TTO	**SG versus RS**	**TTO versus RS**
Study samples with significant differences (N)*	45†	28	38	32

*Statistical tests based on means, SDs, and *N*s reported in studies, and do not account for the fact that the same patients responded to all the three instruments.

†Standard deviations are not available in one study.

When we look within individual samples of participants, on the other hand, we see large numbers of samples with significant differences ($p < 0.05$) between all the three methods. They range from a low of 28 out of 45 significant differences (62%) for the comparison of standard gambles and time trade-offs to a high of 38 out of 45 (84%) for the comparison of standard gambles and rating scales.

These findings differ somewhat from those of Tengs and Lin [71,72]. In their meta-analyses of mixed sets of respondents – i.e., patients, caregivers, providers, and members of the community – who rated current health or disease scenarios for HIV [71] or stroke [72], Tengs and Lin found that time trade-offs appeared to yield the highest preference scores. Standard gamble preference scores were generally 0.1 lower than those for time trade-offs, but in neither case was the difference statistically significant ($p = 0.16$ for HIV and $p = 0.08$ for stroke). Finally, rating scale scores were −0.02 less than those for standard gambles when HIV was rated ($p = 0.001$ compared to time trade-off; NS compared to standard gamble) and were −0.11 lower when stroke was rated ($p = 0.006$ compared to time trade-off; p-value not explicitly reported compared to standard gambles).

4.3.8. Comparison of prescored instruments and direct elicitation methods

Finally, a number of studies have compared preference scores derived from prescored instruments and from direct elicitation methods. As with the previous comparison, we can weight the results from each sample by its number of participants or we can average across the sample means. In either case, as can be seen in Table 4.5, the results derived by use of the prescored instruments are more similar to those derived by use of rating scales than they are to those

Table 4.5 Comparison of preference scores derived by use of the three direct elicitation methods and the three prescored instruments

Average scores for each instrument and method

	Samples, (*N*)	Participants, (*N*)	Standard gamble	Time trade-off	Rating scale	Prescored instrument
Weighted average						
EQ-5D	11	1567	0.89	0.87	0.76	0.70
HUI2	7	293	0.88	0.82	0.75	0.77
HUI3	11	649	0.91	0.83	0.75	0.73
Simple average						
EQ-5D	11	1567	0.87	0.86	0.71	0.70
HUI2	7	293	0.88	0.82	0.76	0.80
HUI3	11	649	0.90	0.82	0.76	0.76

Number of studies with statistically significant differences between preference scores derived by direct elicitation and by prescored instruments*

	Samples, (*N*)	Participants, (*N*)	Standard gamble	Time trade-off	Rating scale
EQ-5D	11	1567	9	11	7
HUI2	7	293	3	4	4
HUI3	11	649	8	7	4

*Statistical tests based on means, SDs, and *N*s reported in studies, and do not account for the fact that the same patients responded to all the three instruments.

derived by use of either the standard gamble or the time trade-off. Also, as with the previous comparison, this result is not as strong when we look at individual samples of participants. In this case, the HUI3 continues to have stronger associations with the rating scale than it does with either the standard gamble or time trade-off, but for the HUI2 there is little statistical evidence about differences in strength of association.

It is not exactly clear what we should make of these relationships. On the one hand, there is the general recommendation that measures of preference used in economic evaluations should be derived from the general public [1]. That is one reason for the use of prescored instruments, because they are administered to patients but the resulting scores are derived from the general public. On the other hand, there is some evidence that patients' preferences for their health are higher than are the general public's when asked to rate scenarios that mirror the patients' health [71,73–77], although Neumann *et al.* [78] have reported that the evidence is not conclusive [72,79–82]. But here we have evidence that what is sometimes considered the least preferred method for the direct elicitation of preferences is certainly no worse at reproducing the results of prescored instruments than are the other direct elicitation methods, and in fact may do better than these other methods.

4.3.9. **Choice between instruments/methods**

So returning to the question of choice of instrument that we posed in our discussion of prescored instruments, what are we to make of these findings? After reading our review of the literature, you may have formed your own opinion about which method is best for eliciting preferences. That opinion might be based on theory, ease of use, or empirical relationships between the different scores.

Nothing we have said runs counter to the recommendation that we should measure both the general public's and patients' preferences in trials. But our review has not led us to strong conclusions about which methods are best for these measurements. Our interpretation of this literature is that getting preferences exactly right is complicated, both because human preferences are so variable and have so many determinants and because all the techniques used to measure preferences are flawed. We are concerned that many of the "recommendations" from commentators seem to be based on theories that ignore this complexity and these flaws. Yes, it would again be easy for us to recommend that you assess the sensitivity of your results to the source of preference scores, but we again recognize that such a strategy is costly. In sum, we are uncomfortable with strong recommendations about the adoption of specific methods or instruments.

4.4. **Constructing QALYs by use of preference scores**

Once we have administered one of these methods repeatedly to a study participant, how do we go about constructing a measure of QALYs? Suppose we administer the HUI2 to an individual every 3 months for 2 years, and she provides the responses depicted in Table 4.6. The right-most column reports the resulting scores from the HUI2's utility scoring rule. These scores are plotted in Fig. 4.4. QALYs are derived by estimating the area under this curve; discounted QALYs are derived by discounting the area under this curve. See Box 4.1 for details.

4.5. **Frequency of elicitation**

Preferences are usually measured for all participants of trials at prescheduled intervals, for example baseline and semi-annually thereafter. Other designs

Table 4.6 Hypothetical responses to the HUI2 measured quarterly for 2 years*

Month	SE	MO	EM	CO	SC	PN	FE	Score
0	1	2	2	1	1	1	1	0.896
3	1	2	2	1	1	1	1	0.896
6	1	3	3	1	2	3	1	0.535
9	1	3	3	1	1	2	1	0.640
12	1	2	3	1	1	2	1	0.748
15	1	2	2	1	1	2	1	0.868
18	1	2	2	1	1	1	1	0.896
21	1	2	2	1	1	1	1	0.896
24	1	2	2	1	1	1	1	0.896

*SE: sensory; MO: mobility; EM: emotion; CO: cognition; SC: self-care; PN: pain; and FE: fertility. Table entries represent levels for each domain. Lower levels represent better function (e.g., 1,1,1,1,1,1,1 represents full functioning).

that yield unbiased results include assessment at random intervals (following designs like those sometimes used in pharmacokinetics studies) or random assignment to assessment intervals. For example, one might measure preferences for a 25% sample of participants every month, such that, including the baseline measure, every participant has five measurements during the first

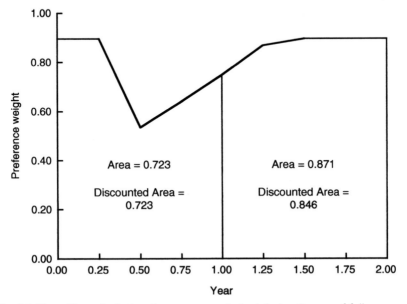

Fig. 4.4 Plot of hypothetical preference scores derived during 2 years of follow-up.

Box 4.1 Calculation of QALYS

Suppose you measured QALYs nine times during a 2-year trial, at baseline and quarterly thereafter. We estimate the area under the curve by use of time-weighted averages of the preference scores measured at the beginning and end of each measurement period (e.g., quarter). For example, in the case we have described, we can sum the values at the beginning and end of each quarter, divide by two (to estimate the average preference score during the quarter), and multiply times 0.25 (because 3 months represents a quarter of a year). Table B4.1.1 shows these steps. In the example, the participant experienced 1.594 undiscounted QALYs out of a possible two undiscounted QALYs during the 2 years of follow-up.

Discounted QALYs are calculated by discounting the QALYs obtained in each year of follow-up by the appropriate discount rate (see equation below). In the example, this patient experiences 1.568 discounted out of a possible 1.971 discounted QALYs during the 2 years of follow-up.

$$\frac{0.723}{1.03^0} + \frac{0.871}{1.03^1} = 1.569$$

Inspection of Table B4.1.1 indicates that if all intervals are of equal length, there is an easier way to calculate annual QALYs. For a given period of time, for example the first year of the trial, we multiply the first and last measurements times 0.5 and times the fraction of the year represented by the measurement (in this case 0.25); we multiply all other measurements

Table B4.1.1 Calculating QALYs as a function of the preference score at the beginning and end of each quarter of observation

Quarter	Calculation		QALYs
0–3 months	$(0.896+0.896) \times 0.5 \times 0.25$	=	0.224
3–6 months	$(0.896+0.535) \times 0.5 \times 0.25$	=	0.178875
6–9 months	$(0.535+0.640) \times 0.5 \times 0.25$	=	0.146875
9–12 months	$(0.640+0.748) \times 0.5 \times 0.25$	=	0.1735
Total, year 1			0.723
12–15 months	$(0.748+0.868) \times 0.5 \times 0.25$	=	0.202
15–18 months	$(0.868+0.896) \times 0.5 \times 0.25$	=	0.2205
18–21 months	$(0.896+0.896) \times 0.5 \times 0.25$	=	0.224
21–24 months	$(0.896+0.896) \times 0.5 \times 0.25$	=	0.224
Total, year 2		=	0.871
2-year total			1.594

Box 4.1 Calculation of QALYS *(continued)*

within the interval times the fraction of the year represented by the measurement. In the current example, for the first year, we multiply measurements the measurements at 3, 6, and 9 months times 0.25 and we continue to multiply measurements at 0 and 12 months by 0.5×0.25. The resulting estimates of QALYs for the first and second years are given below:

Year 1

$$(0.896 \times 0.5 \times 0.25) + (0.896 \times 0.25) + (0.535 \times 0.25) +$$
$$(0.640 \times 0.25) + (0.748 \times 0.5 \times 0.25) = 0.723$$

Year 2

$$(0.748 \times 0.5 \times 0.25) + (0.868 \times 0.25) + (0.896 \times 0.25) +$$
$$(0.896 \times 0.25) + (0.896 \times 0.5 \times 0.25) = 0.871$$

Discounting proceeds in the same manner as above.

---

year, but the measurements are not all at the same intervals. A design that will lead to biased results, on the other hand, is one that purposively samples when a clinical outcome occurs, such as onset of myocardial infarction during follow-up.

How frequently should QALYs be assessed in trials? The answer depends in part on one's beliefs about how rapidly changes are expected in preference, the likely duration of these changes, the length of follow-up, and the resources available for data collection. For trials that last several years, we routinely recommend assessing preferences at least twice a year. In a recent long-term trial, we recommended quarterly assessment during the first year of follow-up, because we expected early onset of improvements in quality of life and we hypothesized that improvement would continue for a number of months before reaching a plateau. Thereafter we measured preferences semi-annually. On the other hand, if, for example, you are involved with a long-term follow-up study (e.g., like those conducted at the end of the Diabetes Control and Complications Trial or the Diabetes Prevention Program) and if resources are limited, you might switch to annual follow-up, particularly if clinical measures are being assessed only once a year.

4.6. **The role of responsiveness in instrument selection**

The last topic we discuss in this chapter is the role of responsiveness in the choice of preference assessment instruments. To borrow from biblical phrasing[1] the fundamental principle of responsiveness theory is: instruments should be responsive when they should be responsive; they should not be responsive when they should not be responsive.

This principle would be simple to employ in the selection of preference assessment instruments if we had a gold standard for the assessment of change in preference, for example an implantable electrode that directly measured utilities. Greater responsiveness would be a sign of criterion validity that should directly influence our choice of instrument. Unfortunately, the electrode is mythical. Rather than having a criterion validity standard, we assess responsiveness of preference measures by use of convergent validity standards: do changes in preference assessment scores correlate – as measured by correlation, effect size, or probability of making a transition – with changes in other measures that we believe are correlated with preference?

The problem that arises when we do not have a criterion validity standard is that we lose the ability to rate the quality of preference assessment instruments based simply on the magnitude of their responsiveness. As we noted in our discussion of choice between prescored instruments above, health preference is not the same as health status. Thus, too high a correlation between changes in preference and function scores may be an indication that the preference instrument is measuring functional status rather than preference.

While these principles are well known, greater responsiveness has always had an allure to those considering the choice of instruments. This allure is illustrated in an elegant study of responsiveness by Marra *et al.* [37]. The authors evaluated the responsiveness of the EQ-5D, HUI2, HUI3, and the SF-6D in a sample of patients with rheumatoid arthritis (RA). They reported that "the EQ-5D appeared to be most responsive to disease worsening but not to improvement"; the HUI3 and SF-6D conversely "were superior in detecting improvement". They concluded, "Thus, in RA clinical trial situations where a known effective intervention is to be applied and there is a large probability of positive change, the SF-6D and the HUI3 would be superior to other instruments" (p. 1342). The authors do not say so, but by implication, they would also conclude that if the larger probability was that the intervention would slow worsening, the EQ-5D would be the superior instrument.

There are multiple problems with these statements. In terms of technical issues, first, there were no stated prior hypotheses about their finding that the EQ-5D would respond better to worsening, and the HUI3 and SF-6D would respond better to improvement, and the findings were the result of multiple

---

[1] "I will be gracious to whom I will be gracious, and will show mercy on whom I will show mercy." (Exodus 33:19).

comparisons (four instruments were compared to two measures of change which were subdivided into three categories (improve, remain the same, worsen). Thus, the probability that we would see this same pattern of results in a replication of this study is actually quite low.

Second, even if the findings were correct, they most likely would apply only to the particular spectrum of disease severity among the patients who were included in the authors' study. It is highly unlikely that the EQ-5D is only responsive to decrements in health across all levels of severity of disease and that the HUI3 and SF-6D are only responsive to improvements across this same range. For example, Conner-Spady and Suarez-Almazor [29] reported that in a mixed sample of rheumatology patients (51% RA), those patients who reported a clinical improvement had larger changes in their EQ-5D scores than their HUI3 scores and those who reported a clinical decrement had smaller changes in their EQ-5D scores than their HUI3 scores.

But the deeper problem with the authors' conclusions is theoretical, not technical. There is a well-recognized pattern of responsiveness across the spectrum of quality of life measures. Disease-specific measures are generally more responsive than generic measures (although not all instruments nor in all diseased populations) [83], and generic profile measures (e.g., the SF-36) are generally more responsive than generic preference-weighted quality of life instruments. Unless and until we know how much the less-responsive preference-weighted instruments should change in the face of changes in the more-responsive disease-specific health status questions, we cannot be sure that the apparently greater responsiveness to improvement observed for the HUI3 and SF-6D recommends or counts against these instruments.

This mistake of associating "most responsive" instrument with "best instrument" is not limited to these authors, and had their article not illustrated the point so well, we would have preferred not to have identified any single group of researchers. In fact, this mistake is a common one. In studies where we have compared instruments, our co-investigators routinely have wondered why we have not always recommended the most responsive instrument, even when there were theoretical or other reasons why we believed the less-responsive instrument was the better one.

Part of the problem stems from confusion about the classic dictum in trial design that one should not adopt instruments that are not responsive. This dictum does not imply we should not do equivalence studies. It relates to the half of the fundamental principle of responsiveness that states that instruments should be responsive when they should be responsive, and specifically to the instrument's capacity to be responsive, not to whether it is responsive in a particular sample of patients.

The difficulty we face is that across a wide range of major diseases we know that preference assessment instruments are responsive, although we also know they are not as responsive as disease-specific instruments. Thus, when we encounter a disease or a sample of patients where they do not appear to be, we do not know whether the instrument is at fault or whether, compared to cancers, myocardial infarctions, and chronic obstructive pulmonary disease, changes in the disease in question simply do not have a substantial impact on how patients trade-off life expectancy and quality of life.

In conclusion, instruments should be responsive when we believe that the changes in the disease we are studying are large enough to affect how patients trade-off quantity and quality of life. But as with our evaluation of the discriminating ability of the prescored instruments above, higher correlations between change in scores and convergent validity criteria do not necessarily indicate a better instrument. Responsiveness is simply another characteristic that weighs into the selection of preference assessment instruments.

4.7. **Summary**

We have reviewed the two most common approaches for assessing QALYs in trials, use of prescored instruments and direct elicitation. We described the EQ-5D, the HUI2 and the HUI3, three of the most commonly used prescored instruments; we also described the standard gamble, the time trade-off, and the rating scale, three of the most commonly used methods for directly eliciting preference scores.

We found evidence from a large number of studies that the HUI2 yields preference scores that are significantly different than the scores from the EQ-5D and the HUI3. Evidence was more mixed about whether HUI3 and EQ-5D scores differ. In one large study, mean EQ-5D scores were significantly lower than mean HUI3 scores, whereas in another large study the reverse was true. The existence of differences between the instruments' scores and the fact that there is little if any evidence that supports the superiority of one instrument over another is problematic, in that they all should be measuring the same construct and thus should yield scores that are indistinguishable from one another.

When we averaged across multiple studies, we found that mean scores from standard gambles and time trade-offs were more similar to each other than they were to rating scale scores. However, when we looked within individual studies, there was substantial evidence that all three methods' scores differed significantly. When we compared scores from prescored instruments with directly elicited scores, we found the directly elicited scores were more similar to rating scale scores than they were to scores from either the standard gamble or the time trade-off.

In sum, when we consider criteria such as appropriateness, reliability and validity, responsiveness, and practicality, our review has not led us to strong conclusions about which of the prescored instruments or direct elicitation methods are best for assessing preferences for health. This conclusion is in accordance with the Panel on Cost Effectiveness' research recommendation that "preference results obtained from techniques employing simpler methods... should be compared to results obtained using the more traditional methods of time tradeoff and standard gamble" (Chapter 4, Research Recommendation 4, p. 123 [1]).

References

1. Gold MR, Siegel JE, Russell LB, Weinstein MC (eds). *Cost-Effectiveness in Health and Medicine*. Oxford: Oxford University Press, 1996.

2. Lundberg L, Johannesson M, Silverdahl M, Hermansson C, Lindberg M. Quality of life, health-state utilities and willingness to pay in patients with psoriasis and atopic eczema. *Br J Dermatol*. 1999; 141: 1067–75.

3. Sevy S, Nathanson K, Schechter C, Fulop G. Contingency valuation and preferences of health states associated with side effects of antipsychotic medications in schizophrenia. *Schizophr Bull*. 2001; 27: 643–52.

4. Stavem K. Association of willingness to pay with severity of chronic obstructive pulmonary disease, health status and other preference measures. *Int J Tuberc Lung Dis*. 2002; 6: 542–9.

5. Sach TH, Whynes DK, O'Neill C, O'Donoghue GM, Archbold SM. Willingness-to-pay for pediatric cochlear implantation. *Int J Pediatr Otorhinolaryngol*. 2004; 68: 91–9.

6. Leighl NB, Tsao WS, Zawisza DL, Nematollahi M, Shepherd FA. A willingness-to-pay study of oral epidermal growth factor tyrosine kinase inhibitors in advanced non-small cell lung cancer. *Lung Cancer* 2006; 51: 115–21.

7. Diener A, O'Brien B, Gafni A. Health care contingent valuation studies: a review and classification of the literature. *Health Econ*. 1998; 7: 313–26.

8. Klose T. The contingent valuation method in health care. *Health Policy* 1999; 47; 97–123.

9. Olsen JA, Smith RD. Theory versus practice: a review of 'willingness-to-pay' in health and health care. *Health Econ*. 2001; 10: 39–52.

10. McNeil BJ, Weichselbaum R, Pauker SG. Speech and survival. Tradeoffs between quality and quantity of life in laryngeal cancer. *NEJM*. 1981; 305: 982–7.

11. Rasanen P, Roine E, Sintonen H, Semberg-Konttinen V, Ryynanen OP, Roine R. Use of quality-adjusted life years for the estimation of effectiveness of health care: a systematic literature review. *Int J Technol Assess Health Care* 2006; 22: 235–41.

12. The EuroQol Group. EuroQol – a new facility for the measurement of health-related quality of life. *Health Policy* 1990; 16: 199–208.

13. The EuroQol Group. Cross-cultural adaptation of health measures. *Health Policy* 1991; 19: 33–44.

14. Torrance GW, Feeny DH, Furlong WJ, Barr RD, Zhang Y, Wang Q. Multi-attribute preference functions for a comprehensive health status classification system: Health Utilities Index Mark 2. *Med Care* 1996; 34: 702–22.

15. Feeny D, Furlong W, Torrance GW, Goldsmith CH, Zhu Z, Depauw S, Denton M, Boyle M. Multiattribute and single-attribute utility functions for the Health Utilities Index Mark 3 System. *Med Care* 2002; 40: 113–28.

16. Brazier J, Roberts J, Deverill M. The estimation of a preference-based measure of health from the SF-36. *J Health Econ.* 2002; 21: 271–92.

17. Kaplan RM, Anderson JP, Wu AW, Mathews WC, Kozin F, Orenstein D. The quality of well-being scale. *Med Care* 1989; 27: S27–S43.

18. Sintonen H, Pekurinen M. *A fifteen-dimensional measure of health-related quality of life (15D) and its applications.* In Quality of Life Assessment. Key Issues in the 1990s, edited by S.R. Walker and R. Rosser. Dordrecht: Kluwer Academic Publishers, pp. 185–95, 1993.

19. Rosser R, Kind P. A scale of valuations of states of illness: is there a social consensus? *Int J Epidemiol.* 1978; 7: 347–358.

20. Rosser R, Cottee M, Rabin T, Selai C. *Index of health-related quality-of-life.* In Measures of the Quality of Life, edited by A. Hopkins. London: Royal College of Physicians, pp. 81–9, 1992.

21. Dolan P. Modeling valuations for the EuroQol health states. *Med Care* 1997; 35: 1095–108.

22. Johnson JA, Coons SJ, Ergo A, Szava-Kovats G. Valuation of EuroQol (EQ-5D) health states in an adult US sample. *Pharmacoeconomics* 1998; 13: 421–33.

23. Polsky D, Willke R, Scott K, Schulman K, Glick HA. A comparison of scoring weights for the EuroQol derived from patients and the general public. *Health Econ.* 2001; 10: 27–37.

24. Torrance GW. Utilities the easy way. The Synergy Innovator 1997; 1: 1.

25. McCabe C, Stevens K, Roberts J, Brazier J. Health state values for the HUI 2 descriptive system: results from a UK survey. *Health Econ.* 2005; 14: 231–44.

26. Blanchard C, Feeny D, Mahon JL, Bourne R, Rorabeck C, Stitt L, Webster-Bogaert S. Is the Health Utilities Index responsive in total hip arthroplasty patients? *J Clin Epidemiol.* 2003; 56: 1046–54.

27. Bosch JL, Hunink MGM. Comparison of the Health Utilities Index Mark 3 (HUI3) and the EuroQol EQ-5D in patients treated for intermittent claudication. *Qual Life Res.* 2000; 9: 591–601.

28. Chong CAKY, Gulamhussein A, Heathcote EJ, Lilly L, Sherman M, Naglie G, Krahn M. Health-state utilities and quality of life in hepatitis C patients. *Am J Gastroenterol.* 2003; 98: 630–8.

29. Conner-Spady B, Suarez-Almazor ME. Variation in the estimation of quality-adjusted life-years by different preference-based instruments. *Med Care* 2003; 41: 791–801.

30. Feeny D, Furlong W, Saigalf S, Sun J. Comparing directly measured standard gamble scores to HUI2 and HUI3 utility scores: group- and individual-level comparisons. *Soc Sci Med.* 2004; 58: 799–809.

31. Luo N, Johnson JA, Shaw JW, Feeny D, Coons SJ. Self-reported health status of the general adult U.S. population as assessed by the EQ-5D and Health Utilities Index. *Med Care* 2005; 43: 1078–86.

32. Marra CA, Woolcott JC, Kopec JA, Shojania K, Offer R, Brazier JE, Esdaile JM, Anis AH. A comparison of generic, indirect utility measures (the HUI2, HUI3, SF-6D, and the EQ-5D) and disease-specific instruments (the RAQoL and the HAQ) in rheumatoid arthritis. *Soc Sci Med*. 2005; 60: 1571–82.

33. McDonough CM, Grove MR, Tosteson TD, Lurie JD, Hilibrand AS, Tosteson AN. Comparison of EQ 5D, HUI, and SF 36 derived societal health state values among spine patient outcomes research trial (SPORT) participants. *Qual Life Res*. 2005; 14: 1321–32.

34. Neumann PJ, Sandberg EA, Araki SS, Kuntz KM, Feeny D, Weinstein MC. A comparison of HUI2 and HUI3 utility scores in Alzheimer's disease. *Med Decis Making* 2000; 20: 413–22.

35. Siderowf A, Ravina B, Glick HA. Preference based quality of life in patients with Parkinson's disease. *Neurology* 2002; 59: 103–8.

36. Suarez-Almazor ME, Kendall C, Johnson JA, Skeith K, Vincent D. Use of health status measures in patients with low back pain in clinical settings. Comparison of specific, generic and preference based instruments. *Rheumatology* 2000; 39: 783–90.

37. Marra CA, Rashidi AA, Buh D, Kopec JA, Abrahamowicz M, Esdaile JM, Brazier ME, Fortin PR, Anis AH. Are indirect utility measures reliable and responsive in rheumatoid arthritis patients? *Qual Life Res*. 2005; 14: 1333–44.

38. Lubetkin EI, Gold MR. Areas of decrement in health-related quality of life (HRQL): Comparing the SF-12, EQ-5D, and HUI 3. *Qual Life Res*. 2003; 12: 1059–67.

39. Morimoto T, Fukui T. Utilities measured by rating scale, time trade-off, and standard gamble: review and reference for health care professionals. *J Epidemiol*. 2002; 12: 160–78.

40. von Neumann J, Morgenstern O. Theory of Games and Economic Behavior. New York: Wiley, 1953.

41. Drummond MF, Sculpher MJ, Torrance GW, O'Brien BJ, Stoddart GL. *Methods for the Economic Evaluation of Health Care Programmes*, 3rd ed. Oxford: Oxford University Press, 2005.

42. Torrance GW, Thomas WH, Sackett DL. A utility maximization model for evaluation of health care programs. *Health Serv Res*. 1972; 7: 118—33.

43. Green C, Brazier J, Deverill M. Valuing health-related quality of life. *Pharmacoeconomics* 2000; 17: 151–65.

44. Happich M, Lengerke Tv. Valuing the health state "tinnitus": differences between patients and the general public. *Hear Res*. 2005; 207: 50–8.

45. Lenert LA, Cher DJ, Goldstein DK, Bergen MR, Garber A. The effect of search procedures on utility elicitations. *Med Decis Making* 1998; 18: 76–83.

46. Hammerschmidt T, Zeitler H-P, Gulich M, Leidl R. A comparison of different strategies to collect standard gambles. *Med Decis Making* 2004; 24: 493–503.

47. Chang WT, Collins ED, Kerrigan CL. An internet-based utility assessment of breast hypertrophy. *Reconstr Surg*. 2001; 108: 370–7.

48. Percy ME, Llewellyn-Thomas H. Assessing preferences about the DNR order: does it depend on how you ask? *Med Decis Making* 1995; 15: 209–16.

49. Tsevat J, Goldman L, Lamas GA, Pfeffer MA, Chapin CC, Connors KF, Lee TH. Functional status versus utilities in survivors of myocardial infarction. *Med Care* 1991; 29: 1153–9.

50. Verhoef LCG, De Haan AFJ, Van Daal WAJ. Risk attitude in gambles with years of life: empirical support for prospect theory. *Med Decis Making* 1994; 14: 194–200.

51. Franic DM, Pathak DS, Gafni A. Are health states "timeless"? A case study of an acute condition: post-chemotherapy nausea and vomiting. *J Eval Clin Pract*. 2003; 9: 69–82.

52. Stiggelbout AM, Kiebert GM, Kievit J, Leer JW, Habbema JD, De Haes JC. The "utility" of the time trade-off method in cancer patients: feasibility and proportional trade-off. *J Clin Epidemiol*. 1995; 48: 1207–14.

53. Bala MV, Wood LL, Zarkin GA, Norton EC, Gafni A, O'Brien BJ. Are health states "time-less"? The case of the standard gamble method. *J Clin Epidemiol*. 1999; 52: 1047–53.

54. Loomes G, McKenzie L. The use of QALYs in health care decision making. *Soc Sci Med*. 1989; 28: 299–308.

55. Dolan P, Gudex C, Kind P, Williams A. Valuing health states: a comparison of methods. *J Health Econ*. 1996; 15: 209–31.

56. Glasziou PP, Bromwich S, Simes RJ, for the AUS-TASK Group. Quality of life six months after myocardial infarction treated with thrombolytic therapy. *Med J Aust*. 1994; 161: 532–6.

57. Nease Jr. RF, Tsai R, Hynes LM, Littenberg B. Automated utility assessment of global health. *Qual Life Res*. 1996; 5: 175–82.

58. Mrus JM, Sherman KE, Leonard AC, Sherman SN, Mandell KL, Tsevat J. Health values of patients coinfected with HIV/hepatitis C. Are two viruses worse than one? *Med Care* 2006; 44: 158–66.

59. Lenert LA. The reliability and internal consistency of an internet-capable computer program for measuring utilities. *Qual Life Res*. 2000; 9: 811–17.

60. Lenert LA, Sturley A, Watson ME. iMPACT3: internet-based development and admin-istration of utility elicitation protocols. *Med Decis Making* 2002; 22: 464–72.

61. Goldstein MK, Miller DE, Davies S, Garber AM. Quality of life assessment software for computer-inexperienced older adults: multimedia utility elicitation for activities of daily living. *Proc AMIA Symp*. 2002; 295–9.

62. van Wijck EEE, Bosch JL, Hunink MGM. Time-tradeoff values and standard-gamble utilities assessed during telephone interviews versus face-to-face interviews. *Med Decis Making* 1998; 18: 400–5.

63. Essink Bot ML, Bonsel GJ, van der Maas PJ. Valuation of health states by the general public: feasibility of a standardized measurement procedure. *Soc Sci Med*. 1990; 31: 1201–6.

64. Silvertssen E, Field NB, Abdelnoor M. Quality of life after open heart surgery. *Vasc Surg*. 1994; 28: 581–8.

65. Ross PL, Littenberg B, Fearn P, Scardino PT, Karakiewicz PI, Kattan MW. Paper standard gamble: a paper-based measure of standard gamble utility for current health. *Int J Technol Assess Health Care* 2003; 19: 135–47.

66. Littenberg B, Partilo S, Licata A, Kattan MW. Paper standard gamble: the reliability of a paper questionnaire to assess utility. *Med Decis Making* 2003; 23: 480–8.

67. Woloshin S, Schwartz LM, Moncur M, Gabriel S, Tosteson ANA. Assessing values for health: numeracy matters. *Med Decis Making* 2001; 21: 382–90.

68. Johannesson M, Jonsson B, Karlsson G. Outcome measurement in economic evaluation. *Health Econ*. 1996; 5: 279–96.

69. Brazier J, Deverill M, Green C, Harper R, Booth A. A review of the use of health status measures in economic evaluation. NHS R&D HTA programme. *Health Technol Assess* 1999; 3(9).

70. Parkin D, Devlin N. Is there a case for using visual analog scale valuations in cost-utility analysis? *Health Econ*. 2006; 15: 653–64.

71. Tengs TO, Lin TH. A meta-analysis of utility estimates of HIV/AIDS. *Med Decis Making* 2002; 22: 475–81.

72. Tengs TO, Lin TH. A meta-analysis of quality-of-life estimates for stroke. *Pharmacoeconomics* 2003; 21: 191–200.

73. Calhoun EA, Fishman DA, Lurain JR, Welshman EE, Bennett CL. A comparison of ovarian cancer treatments: analysis of utility assessments of ovarian cancer patients, at-risk population, general population, and physicians. *Gynecol Oncol* 2004; 93: 164–9.

74. Epstein AM, Hall JA, Tognetti J, Son LH, Conant Jr. L. Using proxies to evaluate quality of life. Can they provide valid information about patients' health status and satisfaction with medical care? *Med Care* 1989; 27: S91–8.

75. Gabriel SE, Kneeland TS, Melton 3rd LJ, Moncur MM, Ettinger B, Tosteson AN. Health-related quality of life in economic evaluations for osteoporosis: whose values should we use? *Med Decis Making* 1999; 19: 141–8.

76. Prosser LA, Kuntz KM, Bar-Or A, Weinstein MC. Patient and community preferences for treatments and health states in multiple sclerosis. *Mult Scler*. 2003; 9: 311–19.

77. Sackett DL, Torrance GW. The utility of different health states as perceived by the general public. *J Chronic Dis*. 1978; 31: 697–704.

78. Neumann PJ, Goldie SJ, Weinstein MC. Preference-based measures in economic evaluation in health care. *Annu Rev Public Health* 2000; 21: 587–611.

79. Llewellyn-Thomas H, Sutherland HJ, Tibshirani R, Ciamp A, Till JE, Boyd NF. Describing health states: methodologic issues in obtaining values for health states. *Med Care* 1984; 22: 543–52.

80. Patrick DL, Sittampalam Y, Somerville S, Carter W, Bergner M. A cross-sectional comparison of health status values. *Am J Public Health* 1985; 75: 1402–7.

81. Balaban DJ, Sagi PC, Godfarb NI, Nettler S. Weights for scoring the quality of well-being instrument among rheumatoid arthritics: a comparison to general population weights. *Med Care* 1986; 24: 973–80.

82. Revicki DA, Shakespeare A, Kind P. Preferences for schizophrenia-related health states: a comparison of patients, caregivers, and psychiatrists. *Clin Psychopharmacol*. 1996; 11: 101–8.

83. Wiebe S, Guyatt G, Weaver B, Matijevic S, Sidwell C. Comparative responsiveness of generic and specific quality-of-life instruments. *J Clin Epidemiol*. 2003; 56: 52–60.

Chapter 5

Analyzing cost

As we indicated in Chapter 1, once we have quantified the cost and effect of the therapies under study, we need to assess the difference in arithmetic mean cost and effect between the treatment groups and determine whether these differences are likely to be due to chance. In this chapter, we focus on methods for addressing these questions for cost when there is little or no missing or censored cost data; in Chapter 6, we focus on addressing the problems for addressing these questions that are posed by missing or censored cost data.

We do not directly focus on the analysis of effect. When effect is represented by a continuous variable, such as QALYs, many of the same techniques that are used to analyze cost can also be used to analyze effect. When effect is measured as a time to event or a dichotomous variable, one must turn to methods such as survival analysis or logistic regression. We do not address the latter forms of analysis in this book, but would recommend that you consult some of the many texts that describe these analyses, such as Hosmer and Lemeshow's Applied Survival Analysis [1] or Applied Logistic Regression [2].

In what follows, we describe the problems that skewed cost distributions pose to the evaluation of the between-group difference in arithmetic mean cost; explain why this variable is the policy relevant outcome of interest for cost-effectiveness analysis; and discuss the strengths and weaknesses of univariate and multivariable statistical procedures that have commonly been used to estimate and draw inferences about differences in cost.

5.1. The problem

While most introductory discussions of the analysis of continuously scaled data simplify the analysis by assuming that these data are normally distributed, the analysis of health care cost is complicated by a number of common features of these data. First, the cost distribution generally is right skewed with a long, heavy, right tail [3]. Second, methods for addressing this skewness can be further complicated by the fact that cost data can include a substantial proportion of observations with zero cost.

Figure 5.1 provides an example of skewed cost distributions for two treatment groups. For treatment group 0, the arithmetic mean cost is

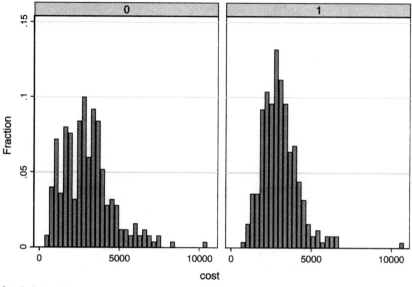

Graphs by treat

Fig. 5.1 Distribution of cost in two treatment groups. A joint skewness and kurtosis test for normality has $p < 0.0001$ that both distributions are nonnormal.

3015 (SD, 1583); the median is 2826, which is less than the arithmetic mean; and the distribution is right-skewed (skewness of 1.04, $p < 0.000$ that rejects the null hypothesis of a symmetric distribution with a skewness of 0). For treatment group 1, the arithmetic mean is 3040 (SD, 1169); the median is 2901; and the distribution is again right-skewed (skewness of 1.53, $p < 0.000$).

There are a number of reasons why cost is routinely characterized by a skewed distribution. First, cost cannot be negative, which places a bound on the lower tail of the distribution (the analog for QALY data is that preference scores cannot exceed 1.0). Cost shares this characteristic with variables such as adult human height that often are considered to be distributed normally; the difference is that cost can and often does equal 0, whereas adult height can not. Second, there is often a nontrivial fraction of study participants that requires substantially more medical services than the norm which make up the long right tail. Third, there usually are a small number of participants – often referred to as outliers – among whom a catastrophic event occurs that leads to a cost that is several standard deviations above the mean. For example, for trials that enroll participants in an outpatient setting, one might observe that most participants are treated solely as outpatients; 15–20% may need routine inpatient care; and 5 participants may require inpatient care that lasts weeks or months.

The distributional problems that arise for cost data are not attributable solely to the few "outliers" in the distribution, but more importantly arise from the nontrivial number of patients who constitute the long right tail. Therefore, approaches such as trimming of outliers – which sometimes are inappropriately used by analysts – do not resolve the problem. To illustrate this impact of thick tails, but not to serve as an endorsement of such data trimming, suppose in our example above that we excluded the six observations that had costs that were three standard deviations above the mean. The arithmetic mean for treatment group 0 would fall from 3015 to 2910, which is still larger than the resulting median of 2813, and the skewness would still be 0.54 ($p = 0.001$). For treatment group 1 the mean, median, and skewness would be 3010, 2885, and 0.71 ($p < 0.000$), respectively.

5.2. **Arithmetic means**

As we have suggested in previous chapters, cost-effectiveness analysis is based on the difference in arithmetic mean cost and the difference in arithmetic mean effect. The arithmetic mean is the important summary statistic from both budgetary and social perspectives [4,5]. From the budgetary perspective, it allows decision makers such as hospital, private insurer, or government to calculate the total cost of adopting a therapy and the total effect received in return for incurring this cost (i.e., arithmetic mean cost times the number of patients treated equals total cost). From the social perspective, it is the minimization of the arithmetic mean cost and maximization of the arithmetic mean effect which yields Kaldor–Hicks social efficiency [6] for the same reasons (i.e., because multiplication of the arithmetic mean times N allows us to determine if those who are made better off by the therapy can potentially compensate those who are made worse off, and yet, still be better off themselves).

Other summary statistics such as median cost – the cost above and below which the cost of half the patients lie – may be useful in describing the data, but they do not provide information about the total cost that will be incurred by treating all patients nor the cost saved by treating patients with one therapy versus another. They, thus, are not associated with social efficiency.

While the mean and median are identical in symmetric distributions like the normal, they differ in skewed distributions. When a distribution is right skewed, the median is smaller than the arithmetic mean; when it is left skewed, the median is larger than the arithmetic mean. The geometric mean cost, which is defined as the Nth root of the product of the observations in the group where N is the number of observations, is always smaller than the mean in the face of non-zero variance and does not permit calculation of the total

Table 5.1 Costs for two treatment groups

Statistic	Treatment group	
	0	1
Mean	3015	3040
SD	1583	1169
Quantiles		
5%	899	1426
25%	1819	2226
50%, Median	2826	2901
75%	3752	3604
95%	6103	5085
Geometric Mean	2601	2836
Mean of Log	7.863486	7.950140

cost by multiplying N times the geometric mean. The data in Fig. 5.1 demonstrate that these statistics need not be equivalent. As shown in Table 5.1, for treatment group 0, the mean, median, and geometric mean are 3015, 2826, and 2601 respectively; for treatment group 1, they are 3040, 2901, and 2836.

Thus, to reiterate, the arithmetic mean and the difference in this mean are the measures we should use for cost-effectiveness analysis in clinical trials. Neither a lack of symmetry nor skewness of the cost distribution changes this fact. Evaluating some other difference, be it a difference in medians or a difference in geometric means, simply because the cost distribution satisfies the assumptions of the tests for these statistics, may be tempting, but does not answer the question we are asking in such trials.

5.3. **Univariate analysis of cost**

In addition to reporting arithmetic mean cost and the difference in this cost, we should routinely report measures of variability such as the standard deviation. When the data are dramatically skewed, it may be helpful to report quantiles of the data. Finally, we should routinely provide an indication of whether the observed differences in arithmetic means are likely to be due to chance. In this section, we discuss univariate analysis of such probability measures.

5.3.1. **Parametric tests of cost on untransformed (raw) scale**

The most common univariate tests of the arithmetic mean are the two-sample t test or – when we are comparing more than two treatments – one-way analysis of variance (ANOVA). One of the assumptions that underlies these tests is that the data are normally distributed. However, in moderately large samples, in samples of similar size and with similar skewness, or samples where skewness is not too extreme, these tests have been shown to be robust to violations of this assumption [4,7–9]. On the other hand, these tests have no requirement about equality of variances across treatment groups, although interpretation depends on whether variances are equal or unequal.

Use of these tests is common in the economic trial literature. Doshi *et al.* [10] found that in 2003, 50% of the published economic assessments based on the analysis of patient level data collected within clinical trials used *t* tests or ANOVA. Nevertheless, because cost data often have a skewness or kurtosis that violate the normality assumption, and because there are no specific thresholds or ranges for sample size or skewness for determining when parametric tests will be reliable, many analysts have rejected these parametric tests. They often have turned to tests of statistics other than the arithmetic mean.

5.3.2. **Nonparametric tests of cost**

One commonly used alternative has been to compare cost by use of nonparametric tests of other characteristics of the distribution that are not as affected by the distribution's nonnormality. Examples of such tests include the Mann–Whitney U (or Wilcoxon rank-sum) test [11,12], the Kolmogorov–Smirnov test [13], and the Kruskall-Wallis test [14].

As we suggested above in the section on arithmetic mean cost, the problem with the use of these tests is that while they tell us that some measure of the cost distribution differs between the treatment groups, such as its shape or location, they do not necessarily tell us that the arithmetic means differ. For example, the Mann–Whitney U test estimates the probability that a randomly selected patient from one treatment group has a higher cost than a randomly selected patient from another treatment group. Thompson and Barber [4] have pointed out that it compares differences in the cost distributions in terms of both shape and location. When one uses a Kolmogorov–Smirnov test, one is testing whether the maximum absolute difference between the cumulative distribution functions for the two treatment groups is the same or different. Finally, the Kruskall–Wallis test is a nonparametric alternative to one-way ANOVA to compare three or more treatment groups. It tests whether the different groups being evaluated were drawn from the same distribution or from distributions with the same median.

Some authors who have adopted nonparametric tests of other characteristics of the distribution have ignored the fact that the resulting *p* values need not be applicable to the arithmetic mean. For example, Doshi *et al.* [10] found that a number of authors reported cost estimates in terms of arithmetic means and the difference in arithmetic means but derived a p value for this difference by use of the Mann–Whitney U test. Furthermore, some studies not only adopted the Mann–Whitney U test, but they reported cost estimates in terms of medians and the difference in the median and did not report the arithmetic mean. Erroneous use of such nonparametric tests does not change the fact that the numerators and denominators of cost-effectiveness ratios, as well as the incremental cost and effect measures used to calculate NMB, should always represent differences in arithmetic mean cost and effect. In other words, while you might decide to compare cost by use of tests like the Mann–Whitney U test, the numerator and denominator of the cost-effectiveness ratio should never be represented as a difference in median cost or effect.

5.3.3. Parametric tests of cost on the transformed scale

When the cost distribution is not normal, some analysts have transformed cost in an attempt to make the distribution of the resulting transformed variable more normal. Examples of such transformations include the logarithmic, square root, or reciprocal transformation. When we make such transformations, we estimate and draw inferences about the difference on the transformed scale, but our fundamental goal is to apply these estimates and inferences to the difference in arithmetic mean of untransformed cost. Thus we need to be concerned about issues that may undermine this applicability.

The logarithmic transformation of cost is widely used in health care cost analysis. The most common reason for its use is that if the resulting distribution of log cost is normal, t tests of log cost may be more efficient than t tests of nonnormally distributed untransformed cost. Some analysts also use a log transformation because the difference in log cost – or the coefficient estimates for explanatory variables in multivariable analysis of log cost – can be interpreted as percentage differences.

Unfortunately, log transformation raises several issues for the analyses of cost. First, when observations have 0 cost, their log cost is undefined. Many researchers address this problem by adding an arbitrary constant such as 1 to all cost observations before taking logs. However, one should always determine whether the magnitude of the arbitrary constant affects one's conclusions, and the presence of a substantial proportion of zeros can make this approach problematic. As we discuss later in this chapter, we should instead analyze such data by use of a two-part model.

Second, transformation does not always yield a normal distribution. For example, Fig. 5.2 shows the results of the log transformation of the cost data that were plotted in Fig. 5.1. For neither treatment group are the resulting log

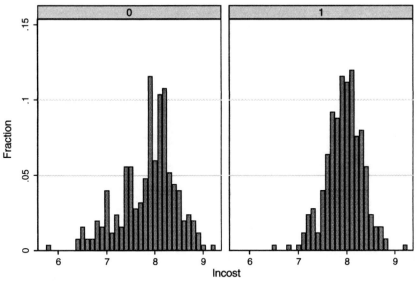

Graphs by treat

Fig. 5.2 Distribution of log cost in the two treatment groups shown in Fig. 5.1. A joint skewness and kurtosis test for normality has $p = 0.002$ and $p = 0.01$ for the two groups, respectively, that the two distributions are nonnormal.

cost data normally distributed. For treatment group 0, the resulting skewness is −0.60 ($p < 0.000$); for treatment group 1, it is −0.30 ($p = 0.05$).

Third, and possibly most important, estimates and inferences about log cost apply more directly to the geometric mean of cost than they do to the arithmetic mean. Table 5.2 illustrates this point with an example of a hypothetical dataset with nine observations, three each in treatment groups 1, 2, and 3.

Estimation

As shown in the top half of the table, the arithmetic mean cost is 30 in group 1. As constructed, the distribution for group 2 is simply a multiple (1.5) of the distribution for group 1, and its arithmetic mean is 45. Group 3 has the same arithmetic mean as group 2, but it has a different variance and its distribution is not a simple multiple of that of group 1. The geometric means equal 24.662 [$(10 \times 30 \times 50)^{1/3}$], 36.993, and 44.247 for the three groups, respectively. The second half of the table shows that exponentiation of the arithmetic mean of the log for each group equals its geometric mean. For example, in group 0, the mean of the logs is 3.205 and $e^{3.205} = 24.662$, in group 2, $e^{3.611} = 36.993$, and in group 3, $e^{3.790} = 44.247$. Thus, simple exponentiation of the mean of the logs

Table 5.2 Cost, log cost, and arithmetic and geometric means

Variable	Group 1	Group 2	Group 3
Observations			
1	10	15	35
2	30	45	45
3	50	75	55
Arithmetic mean	30	45	45
Geometric mean $\sqrt[N]{\prod_{i=1}^{N} Y_i}$	24.662	36.993	44.247
Ratio, geometric/arithmetic mean	0.822	0.822	0.983
Log of arithmetic mean cost	3.401197	3.806662	3.806662
Natural log			
1	2.302585	2.70805	3.555348
2	3.401197	3.806662	3.806662
3	3.912023	4.317488	4.007333
Arithmetic mean of log cost	3.205269	3.610734	3.789781
Standard deviation	0.8224	0.8224	0.2265
$\exp^{(\text{mean ln})}$	24.662	39.993	44.247

yields the geometric mean of cost, which in the presence of variability in cost, is a downward-biased estimate of the arithmetic mean.

If simple exponentiation of the mean of the logs yields the geometric mean of cost, how do we retransform the mean of the logs to obtain an estimate of arithmetic mean cost?

When the distribution of log cost is normal, and when – as in groups 1 and 2 – the treatment groups have a common log variance, we use what we refer to as the common smearing factor proposed by Duan [3]. When the distribution is normal and when the treatment groups have different log variances, or in the multivariable case, there is heteroscedasticity (e.g., treatment groups 2 and 3), we use what we refer to as subgroup-specific smearing factors proposed by Manning [15]. Common and subgroup-specific smearing factors represent the mean of the exponentiated errors in prediction on the log scale, and are described in more detail in Box 5.1. The principal difference between these two sets of smearing factors is whether we calculate a single common smearing factor for the entire sample or whether we calculate multiple, subgroup-specific

Box 5.1 Retransformation of the log of cost

As we have shown, simple exponentiation of the mean of the logs yields the geometric mean of cost, which in the presence of nonzero variance in cost is a downward-biased estimate of the arithmetic mean. One uses a smearing retransformation to obtain estimates of arithmetic mean cost rather than the geometric mean. When the distributions are normal, one uses a common smearing factor when the log variances are equal; one uses subgroup-specific smearing factors when log variances differ.

Common smearing retransformation (groups 1 and 2)

The common smearing factor represents the mean of the exponentiated residuals on the log scale. Equation 5.1.1 defines this factor:

$$\Phi = \frac{1}{N} \sum_{i=1}^{N} e^{\left(z_i - \hat{z}_i\right)} \qquad (5.1.1)$$

where Z_i equals the log of cost for observation i and where, in univariate analysis, $\hat{Z}_i$ equals the treatment group-specific mean of the log (in multivariable analysis, it equals participant i's predicted log cost).

Table B5.1.1 shows the calculation of the common smearing factor for treatment groups 1 and 2. In this experiment, it equals 1.21644. We multiply this smearing factor times the exponential of the mean of the logs

Table B5.1.1 Calculation of the common smearing factor

Group	Observation	ln	$z_i - \hat{z}_i$	$e^{\left(z_i - \hat{z}_i\right)}$
1	1	2.302585	−0.9026834	0.4054801
1	2	3.401197	0.1959289	1.21644
1	3	3.912023	0.7067545	2.027401
Mean, 1	–	3.205269	–	–
2	1	2.708050	−0.9026834	0.4054801
2	2	3.806663	0.1959289	1.216440
2	3	4.317488	0.7067545	2.027401
Mean, 2	–	3.610734	–	–
Smear				**1.21644**

Box 5.1 Retransformation of the log of cost *(continued)*

(24.662 and 36.933) and we obtain estimates of 30 and 45, for the two groups, respectively, which match their arithmetic means.

Subgroup-specific retransformation (groups 2 and 3)

If we were to use a common smearing retransformation in the comparison of groups 2 and 3, we would not observe this equality of the retransformed means and the original arithmetic means. Using the same methods we used to calculate the common smearing factor in Table B5.1.1, the common smearing factor for groups 2 and 3 equals 1.116732 (you may want to try to estimate this factor yourself). When we multiply this smearing factor times the exponential of the mean of the logs (36.933 and 44.247) we obtain estimates of 41.3 and 49.4 for the two groups, respectively, which do not match either group's arithmetic mean.

The reason this problem arises is because the variances/standard deviations of the log of these two groups tend to differ (0.8224 versus 0.2265) (note that the lack of significant difference is due to the small sample sizes we are using in the example). In cases where the standard deviations are not equal, we need to use subgroup-specific smearing factors.

Equation 5.1.2 defines the subgroup-specific smearing factor:

$$\Phi_j = \frac{1}{N_j} \sum_{i=1}^{N_j} e^{\left(z_{ij} - \hat{z}_j\right)} \tag{5.1.2}$$

Table B5.1.2 Calculation of subgroup-specific smearing factors

Group	Observation	ln	$z_i - \hat{z}_i$	$e^{\left(z_i - \hat{z}_i\right)}$
2	1	2.708050	−0.9026834	0.4054801
2	2	3.806663	0.1959289	1.216440
2	3	4.317488	0.7067545	2.027401
Mean, 2	–	3.610734	–	**1.21644**
3	1	3.555348	−0.2344332	0.7910191
3	2	3.806663	0.0168812	1.017025
3	3	4.007333	0.2175519	1.24303
Mean, 3	–	3.535261	–	**1.0170245**

Box 5.1 Retransformation of the log of cost *(continued)*

where Z_{ij} equals the log of cost for observation i in treatment group j and where, in univariate analysis, $\hat{Z}_j$ equals the treatment group-specific mean of the log (as with the common smearing factor, in multivariable analysis, it equals the participant i's predicted log cost).

Table B5.1.2 shows the calculation of the subgroup-specific smearing factors for treatment groups 2 and 3. In this experiment, they equal 1.21644 and 1.0170245, respectively. We multiply these smearing factor times the exponential of the mean of the logs (36.933 and 44.247) and we obtain estimates of 45 for each for the two groups, which again matches their arithmetic means.

---

smearing factors, which in univariate analysis translates into a single smearing factor for each treatment group.

In univariate analysis, subgroup-specific retransformation always provides an unbiased estimate of the arithmetic mean. That is because in univariate analysis subgroup-specific retransformation always yields the sample mean of untransformed cost in each treatment group (see Box 5.1). Common retransformation, on the other hand, need not provide unbiased estimates. That is because even when the distributions pass tests for normality and equal standard deviation, common retransformation will translate small variations in standard deviation, skewness, or kurtosis into differences in the arithmetic mean.

These problems are magnified when the distribution of log cost is not normal. In this case, one cannot rely solely on tests of difference in log variance to determine whether to use common or subgroup-specific smearing retransformation. Difference in variance, nonnormal skewness and kurtosis, and sample size are just some of the factors that play a role in determining which retransformation minimizes error in prediction. Because no simple guideline exists which helps the analyst select the best retransformation, in the face of nonnormality, there is no simple means of knowing which retransformation is appropriate.

Inference

These problems for estimation translate into problems for inference about differences in the arithmetic mean of cost. When one uses a t test to evaluate log cost, the resulting p value has direct applicability to the difference in the log of cost. This p value generally also applies to the difference in the geometric mean of cost (i.e., one sees similar p values for the difference in the log and the difference in the geometric mean).

The p value for the log may or may not be directly applicable to the difference in arithmetic mean of untransformed cost. As with estimation, whether it does or not depends on whether the two distributions of the log are normal and whether they have equal variance and thus standard deviation.

If log cost is normally distributed and if the variances are equal, inferences about the difference in log cost are generally applicable to the difference in arithmetic mean cost. The rationale behind this conclusion can be seen in our example in Table 5.2. When we compare the arithmetic means of groups 1 and 2 in Table 5.2, the standard deviation of the logs is equal (0.8224) for the two groups, which in turn yields a similar ratio between the geometric and arithmetic means (1.21644) in the two groups. Given that the p value for the difference in the log is applicable to the difference in the geometric mean, and given that when the standard deviations of the log are equal between the treatment groups, the groups' arithmetic means are a common multiple of their geometric mean, the p value for the difference in logs will also generally apply to the difference in arithmetic mean cost as well.

On the other hand, if log cost is normally distributed and if the variances are unequal, inferences about the difference in log cost generally will not be applicable to the difference in arithmetic mean cost. For instance, when we compare the arithmetic means of groups 2 and 3, the standard deviation of the logs differs between the two groups, and thus the ratio between the geometric and arithmetic means differs between the two groups. Given that the arithmetic means of the groups are not a common multiple of their geometric means, there is no reason to believe that the p value for the difference in the log – which again is generally applicable to the geometric means of the two groups – necessarily applies to the difference in arithmetic means. In fact, because use of different smearing factors can yield equal arithmetic means of cost when the arithmetic means of log cost differ – or, in even more extreme cases, can yield opposite signs between the difference in arithmetic mean cost and the difference in arithmetic mean log cost – the general expectation is that the p value for the log will not apply to the p value for untransformed cost.

Thus, to conclude, in the presence of inequality of variance on the log scale, comparisons of log cost are not appropriate for drawing statistical inferences about differences in arithmetic mean cost [4,16]. Probably as important, this issue is not unique to the log transformation of cost. As Manning has pointed out, similar problems will arise for any power transformation of cost [15]. Hence, simply adopting a different transformation, e.g., the square root, need not solve the problems we are discussing.

5.3.4. **Nonparametric bootstrap**

If the arithmetic mean is the statistic of interest for decision making, and if the underlying assumptions of parametric tests of this mean are violated, one alternative is to adopt a nonparametric test of arithmetic means. An increasingly popular test of this kind is the nonparametric bootstrap [17,18]. The nonparametric bootstrap procedure, which was developed by Efron, has the advantage of avoiding parametric assumptions about the distribution of cost while allowing inferences about arithmetic mean cost. As a result, the nonparametric bootstrap has been recommended either as a check on the robustness of standard parametric t tests, or as the primary statistical test for making inferences about arithmetic means for small to moderately sized samples of highly skewed cost data [16].

Bootstrap methods assume that the empirical distribution of the data is an adequate representation of the true distribution of the data (other statistical procedures may not need this assumption for their calculation, but all statistical procedures require it for interpretation of their results). Statistical analysis is based on repeatedly sampling from the observed data using common computer software such as Stata, SAS, S-PLUS, and GAUSS.

In brief, we repeatedly randomly draw a sample of size N_j with replacement from each treatment group, where N_j equals the number of study participants in treatment group j. This repetition provides us with a series of resamples or bootstrap datasets, each of which is the equivalent of a repetition of the trial, and all of which have treatment groups of size N_j. These bootstrap samples differ from one another because we have drawn with replacement; had we drawn without replacement, we would have replicated the same trial in each sample. To obtain reliable results in practice, Efron and Tibshirani [17, p. 47] have recommended between 25 and 200 resamples to estimate a bootstrap standard error and at least 1000 resamples to estimate a bootstrap confidence interval [17], although the number needed depends in part on the precision one is seeking.

Within each of the multiple "trials" we calculate the statistic of interest, in this case the difference in arithmetic mean cost. By doing so multiple times, we generate a distribution for the statistic of interest (see the histogram in Fig. 5.3 for the distribution of the difference in arithmetic mean cost for the data shown in Fig. 5.1). This distribution can be used to conduct nonparametric or parametric hypothesis tests, estimate standard errors, and generate nonparametric or parametric confidence intervals. For example, we can use the nonparametric percentile method to derive a one-sided test of the observed difference in the arithmetic mean of 25 (i.e., 3040 − 3015) by determining the fraction of bootstrap replicates in which the difference is below 0 and the

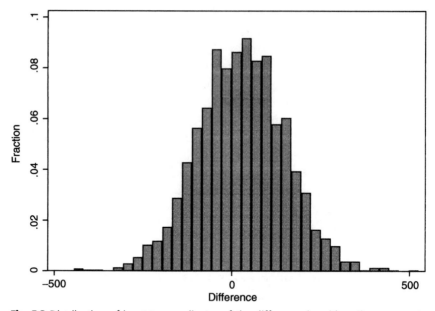

Fig. 5.3 Distribution of bootstrap replicates of the difference in arithmetic mean cost for the two treatment groups shown in Fig. 5.1.

fraction in which it is above 0. In Fig. 5.3, 41.95% fall below 0, in which case the one-sided p value is 0.4195, which we round to 0.42. By convention, we double the one-sided p value if we want a two-sided test (0.84).

We can use this same method to calculate nonparametric confidence intervals by rank ordering the difference in arithmetic mean cost from lowest to highest and identifying the difference in arithmetic mean cost for the replicates that bound the $\alpha/2$ and $1-(\alpha/2)$ percentiles of the distribution of the difference. For example, if there are 1000 bootstrap replicates, and if we wish to construct 95% confidence limits, they are defined by the difference in arithmetic mean cost for the 26th and 975th ordered replicates. In the current example, the 95% confidence interval for the observed difference in arithmetic mean cost ranges from −216 to 269.

For more details on the various bootstrap methods for hypothesis tests and confidence intervals with applications for analysis of cost data from randomized trials, refer to the article by Barber and Thompson [16].

5.3.5. **Comparison of test results**

In Table 5.3, we compare the results from all of the tests we have discussed above in the evaluation of the difference in mean cost for the data shown

Table 5.3 p values from 5 univariate tests of the difference in cost

Test	p value
t test of mean difference, unequal SD	0.84
Nonparametric bootstrap (1,000 replicates)	0.84 (two-tailed)
Mann–Whitney U/Wilcoxon rank-sum	0.37
Kolmogorov–Smirnov	0.002
t test, log of cost difference, unequal SD	0.05
Test of equal standard deviations	0.0000

in Fig. 5.1. While the example and discussion focuses on p values, the same arguments would apply to the calculation of confidence intervals. Both the t test and the nonparametric bootstrap indicate we cannot be 95% confident that arithmetic mean cost differs between the two groups. The Mann–Whitney U test agrees, but as we have already indicated, that is more because the medians (2901 and 2985) are similar than it is because of similar arithmetic means. Support for this last claim comes from the fact that the bootstrapped one-sided p value for the difference in the median is 0.34.

The remaining two tests indicate that cost in the two groups is significantly different. The log cost result is due to the fact that the 235 (2836 − 2601) difference in the geometric means is larger than the difference in either the arithmetic means or medians. In addition, given that the test of equality of standard deviations of log cost fails, we cannot be confident that the p value for the difference in log cost applies to the difference in untransformed cost. The Kolmogorov–Smirnov test result indicates that the cumulative distribution functions of the two treatment groups are statistically different. Inspection of Fig. 5.1 suggests there are differences in skewness and kurtosis in the two groups. The fact that the Kolmogorov–Smirnov test is reported to be sensitive to such differences [19] might explain why its p value is so different from the p value for the Mann–Whitney U test.

Nevertheless, this example demonstrates that the last two tests lead to a very different interpretation for the cost evaluation than do the t test and bootstrap because they are measuring differences in different statistics. If results from the latter two tests were to be used in supporting health care policy decisions, they would be misleading.

5.3.6. **Skewness and small samples**

We would be remiss not to warn readers that in the face of small sample sizes and highly skewed distributions, O'Hagan and Stevens [20] have raised

concerns about whether the sample mean is "necessarily a good basis for inference about the population mean" (p. 34). As they indicate, in these situations,
the sample mean is not robust to skewed data. They argue that a Bayesian
analysis, based on an assumption of a "lognormal distribution of costs produces quite different answers, and a look at the data makes it clear that lognor-
mality is a far more realistic assumption than normality" [20, p. 44]. We leave
it to readers to pursue these methods if they so choose.

To avoid confusion, we also should note that O'Hagan and Stevens' recommendation for use of a Bayesian analysis of the lognormal distribution of cost
differs from the frequentist analysis of log cost that we criticized above.
O'Hagan and Stevens agree that this latter approach addresses the wrong
question (pp. 34, 35).

5.4. Multivariable analysis of cost

The fact that cost data are being collected within a randomized trial does not
mean that use of multivariable models to analyze these data is inappropriate.
In fact, multivariable analysis of cost may be superior to univariate analysis
because by explaining variation due to other causes, it improves the power for
tests of differences between groups. It also facilitates subgroup analyses for
cost-effectiveness, for example for participants with more and less severe
diseases; different countries/centers; etc. Finally, it accounts for potentially
large and influential variations in economic conditions and practice patterns
by provider, center, or country that may not be balanced by randomization in
the clinical trial.

Adoption of multivariable analysis does not, however, avoid the problems
that arise in the univariate analysis of cost. As the recent ISPOR RCT-CEA
Task Force noted, the same distributional problems that affect univariate tests
of cost also affect use of cost as a dependent variable in a multivariable regression analysis [5]. In particular, different multivariable models make different
assumptions. When the assumptions are met, their coefficient estimates will
have desirable properties. When the assumptions that underlie a particular
model are violated, it may produce misleading or problematic coefficient estimates. The two main considerations when comparing models for cost analysis
are (1) bias or consistency and (2) efficiency or precision of the coefficient
estimates of interest, such as those for the variable representing treatment.

5.4.1. Ordinary least squares regression on untransformed cost

Ordinary least squares (OLS) regression on untransformed cost (which in the
absence of other covariates is equivalent to the univariate t test) has been the

most frequently used model for multivariable analysis of cost in randomized clinical trial settings [10]. The advantages of OLS models are that they are easy to implement in any computer software and the incremental cost estimates are easy to calculate, because the coefficient for the treatment indicator provides a direct estimate of the adjusted difference in arithmetic mean cost between the treatment groups. It also yields "best linear unbiased estimates" (see Kennedy [21] for a detailed description of OLS). As with the univariate t test, however, health care data often violate the assumptions underlying OLS.

One assumption that is sometimes violated is that the variance of the error term is constant, referred to as homoscedasticity. When it is not constant, referred to as heteroscedasticity, the resulting coefficients will be unbiased, but the estimates will be inefficient. A second assumption that is often violated is that the error term is normally distributed. This violation affects the variances of the coefficients and undermines the reliability of tests of statistical significance and confidence intervals. Additional problems include that the model results can be highly sensitive to extreme cases; they can be prone to overfitting; and the results may not be robust both in small-to-medium-sized datasets and in large datasets with extreme observations. Thus, while OLS models have been shown to be able to withstand violations of normality – in part because in large samples one can rely on the central limit theorem – these models are difficult to defend in practice.

5.4.2. Ordinary least squares regression on log transformed cost (Log OLS)

In an attempt to overcome problems of heteroscedasticity and skewness of cost data, economists have traditionally used multivariable OLS regression to predict the log of cost. As with the univariate t test of the log, however, results of this regression represent estimates and inferences about log cost, and may not apply to the arithmetic mean of untransformed cost.

Some of the lessons we learned about retransformation after the univariate t test of the log apply equally to retransformation after log OLS. For example, if log cost is normally distributed and there is no evidence of heteroscedasticity, one may be able to use common smearing retransformation and obtain efficiency gains over the estimation of OLS on untransformed cost. As with univariate analysis, however, in the face of heteroscedasticity, the need to use subgroup-specific smearing retransformation indicates that we cannot be confident that the p value for the treatment effect on log cost applies to its effect on the arithmetic mean of cost. In addition, as we discussed in the univariate context, when log cost is not normally distributed, there is no simple way of knowing which retransformation is appropriate, and thus again, no way to know whether the p value for the treatment effect on log cost applies to its effect on the arithmetic mean of cost.

In the multivariable context, there are additional complications for retransformation that do not arise in the univariate context. Some of these complications include the fact that subgroup-specific retransformation is no longer necessarily unbiased in the multivariable setting and that heteroscedasticity among any of the covariates, and not just the treatment group, can pose problems for retransformation.

Thus, while Manning and Mullahy have identified a limited set of situations in which log OLS may be a preferred model [22], in many cases the estimates and inferences derived for log cost will not be applicable to arithmetic mean cost.

5.4.3. Generalized linear models

While the generalized linear model (GLM) was proposed over 30 years ago [23,24], only in recent years has it been slowly making its way into the health economics literature as a means of overcoming shortcomings of OLS and log OLS models [22,25]. These models have the advantage that they directly model both the mean and variance functions on the original scale of cost. To model these functions, we identify a "link function" and a "family" based on the data (see discussion below).

GLM is easily implemented in a number of common statistical software packages. A GLM model with cost y and treatment indicator x is implemented in Stata using the command:

glm y x, family (familyname) link(linkname)

The corresponding language in SAS is:

PROC GENMOD; MODEL Y = X/LINK= linkname DIST = familyname;

The link function specifies the relationship between the mean $(E(y/x))$ and the linear specification of the covariates $(X\beta)$. Examples of link functions include the identity link (e.g., the mean equals $X\beta$), log link, and power links such as square roots. GLM is attractive because the link function directly characterizes how the mean on the untransformed scale is related to the predictors. For example, if one uses a GLM model with a log link, one is modeling the log of arithmetic mean cost (i.e., $\ln(E(y/x))=X\beta$).

GLM with a log link differs from log OLS in part because in log OLS, one does not model the log of arithmetic mean cost but instead models the arithmetic mean of log cost (i.e., $E(\ln(y)/x)=X\beta$). Table 5.2 illustrates that the log of the mean does not equal the mean of log. For example, in group 1, the log

Table 5.4 Comparison of results of GLM and log OLS regression predicting the difference between groups 2 and 3 (Table 5.2)

Variable	Coefficient	SE	Z/T	p value
GLM, gamma family, log link				
Group 3	0.000000	0.405730	0.00	1.000
Constant	3.806662	0.286894	13.27	0.000
Log OLS				
Group 3	0.179048	0.492494	0.36	0.74
Constant	3.610734	0.348246	10.32	0.000

of 30 equals 3.401197 whereas the mean of the logs for the three observations in this treatment group equals 3.205269; for treatment group 2, the log of the mean and the mean of the logs equal 3.806662 and 3.610734, respectively.

Table 5.4 demonstrates this difference in estimation by use of the data for treatment groups 2 and 3 from Table 5.2. As can be seen in Table 5.2, these treatment groups have the same arithmetic mean cost (45) and thus the same log of the arithmetic mean cost (3.806662), but, because of the difference in their variance, have different arithmetic means of log cost (3.610734 versus 3.789781). As seen in Table 5.4, for the GLM, the constant is 3.806662, which equals the log of the mean for group 2. Because the coefficient equals 0, our prediction for group 3 is also 3.806662. Thus, the GLM indicates that the log of the arithmetic means are the same for groups 2 and 3, and it would continue to do so even if the samples were large enough that we would be interested in interpreting the p values.

For the log OLS, the constant is 3.610734, which equals the arithmetic mean of the log for group 2. The coefficient equals 0.1790477, which when added to 3.610734 equals 3.789781, which to the fifth decimal equals the arithmetic mean of the log for group 3. In this example, if the sample sizes were large enough that we would be interested in interpreting the p values, the log OLS would tell us that the arithmetic mean of the log differs between the two treatment groups.

The fact that the GLM predicts the log of the mean rather than the mean of the log leads to several further differences between GLM and log OLS. First, as we have already indicated, because the exponential of the mean of the log represents the geometric, rather than the arithmetic, mean, we need to use a smearing factor to retransform the results of log OLS to predict cost. Because the GLM predicts the log of the mean, it does not suffer from this problem. Simple retransformation of the predicted results from the GLM – without a smearing factor – represents the arithmetic mean. Second, because we do not need to log transform the cost data before estimation of a GLM with a log link, there is no problem with including observations with 0 cost in our analysis.

Finally, unlike OLS and log OLS, GLM allows for heteroscedasticity through a variance structure relating the variance to the mean. This is done by specifying the family which corresponds to a distribution that reflects the mean–variance relationship. For instance, the Gaussian family indicates that the variance is constant. The poisson family indicates that the variance is proportional to the mean; the gamma family assumes variance is proportional to the square of the mean; and the inverse Gaussian or Wald family assumes variance is proportional to the cube of the mean. The modified Parks test is a constructive test for the selection of the appropriate family (see Box 5.2 for details). While misspecification of family results in efficiency losses, it does not affect consistency if the link function and covariates are correctly specified.

Box 5.2 Modified Parks test for generalized linear models

Manning and Mullahy (2001) have proposed the modified Parks Test as a means of identifying the family for a generalized linear model. This test proceeds in five steps, which we have illustrated by use of italicized STATA code.

Step 1. Estimate a GLM regression on sample data assuming any family and link function

```
glm cost treat [covariates], family(gamma) link(log)
```

Step 2. Predict the value of cost (y) on the untransformed scale ($y$hat) and log transform it (ln$y$hat)

```
predict yhat
gen lnyhat = ln(yhat)
```

Step 3. Generate residuals (res) on the untransformed scale and square them

```
gen res = cost-yhat
gen res2=((res)^2)
```

Box 5.2 Modified Parks test for generalized linear models *(continued)*

Step 4. Regress the resulting squared residuals (res2) on the log of the predicted values of y (lnyhat) by use of GLM with a log link, gamma distribution, and robust variance/covariance matrix. By use of the log link, this command is equivalent to regressing the log of the squared residuals on the log of the predicted values of y.

```
glm res2 lnyhat, link(log) family(gamma) robust
```

Step 5. Identify the appropriate family by interpreting the resulting coefficient for lnyhat as shown in Table B5.2.1.

The rationale that underlies this test is that it uses the residuals and predictions on the untransformed scale for costs to estimate and test a very specific form of heteroscedasticity – one where the raw-scale variance is a power function of the raw-scale mean function. The coefficient for lnyhat represents this power function. If it has a value of 0, then it indicates a Gaussian family in which the variance is constant. If it has a value of 1 then it indicates a poisson-like family in which the variance is proportional to the mean; a value of 2 indicates the gamma family in which the variance is proportional to the mean squared; and a value of 3 indicates the inverse Gaussian or Wald family in which the variance is proportional to the cube of the mean.

Table B5.2.1 Interpreting the coefficients from the modified park test

Coefficient	Family	Stata test
0	Gaussian	test lnyhat=0
1	Poisson	test lnyhat=1
2	Gamma	test lnyhat=2
3	Inverse Gaussian or Wald	test lnyhat=3

So far we have presented GLM as if it were superwoman. But as with all statistical approaches, it has its limitations. For example, there is no simple test to identify the appropriate link function for the GLM model, and there has been little guidance in the literature for applied researchers on how to identify the correct link function a priori. The log link has been most commonly used in literature but may not necessarily be the best in all cases. Unlike misspecification of the family, use of the inappropriate link function can impart bias to our results.

One approach that researchers have used to identify the correct link function has been to compare model performance of all permutations of candidate link and variance function using a series of diagnostic tests such as the Pregibon link test [26], which evaluates linearity of the response on the scale of estimation, the modified Hosmer–Lemeshow test [2], which evaluates systematic bias in fit on the raw scale, and Copas test [27], which tests for overfitting and cross validation. As should be apparent, this process can be unwieldy. More recently, Basu and Rathouz [28] have proposed estimation of the link function and family along with other components of the model by use of extended estimating equations (EEE). This approach eliminates the need for the analyst to a priori select family and link functions.

A second potential problem with the GLM is that it can suffer substantial precision losses in datasets with cost distributions having a heavy-tailed log error term, i.e., log-scale residuals have high kurtosis (>3) [22].

Finally, while GLM avoids the problem of retransformation that undermines log OLS, it does not avoid the other complexity of nonlinear retransformations which is faced by all multiplicative models including log OLS, logistic regression, and the like. On the transformed scale, the effect of the treatment group is estimated holding all else equal; however, retransformation (to estimate cost) can reintroduce covariate imbalances. That is because in multiplicative models, the absolute magnitude of the impact of a treatment coefficient such as 0.5 on cost differs depending on the values of the other covariates.

Some have attempted to overcome this last problem by making the retransformation by use of the mean for all covariates excluding the treatment group. The limitation of this approach is that the antilog – or other multiplicative retransformation – of the mean does not equal the mean of the antilogs. Instead we should use the method of recycled predictions. This method creates an identical covariate structure for each treatment group by coding everyone as if they were in the control group (0) and predicting cost for each individual and then coding everyone as if they were in the treatment group (1) and predicting cost for each individual. The difference in the arithmetic mean cost between these two comparisons yields predicted cost that holds all else equal during both model estimation and retransformation.

5.4.4. Alternative multivariable methods

In addition to Basu and Rathouz's EEE [28], Manning *et al.* [29] have proposed regression modeling using the generalized gamma distribution as an alternative estimator. They have argued that this approach will be more robust to violations of distributional assumptions if none of the standard approaches such as GLM or the log OLS are appropriate for the data. Another advantage of the generalized gamma is that it includes several of the standard alternatives as special cases. For example, the ability to use it to estimate OLS with a normal error, OLS for the log normal, the standard gamma and exponential with a log link, and the Weibull allows nested comparisons for alternative estimators.

5.4.5. Special case: analysis of cost data with substantial zeros

An added complication to the analysis of skewed health care cost is the possibility of a substantial number of participants who have incurred no medical cost (the analog for QALY data is the possibility of a substantial number of observations with a preference score of 1.0). In such cases, a single regression model including the zero-cost observations may result in problematic estimates. Also, as we previously indicated, in log OLS models, one can only include these observations if one adds an arbitrary constant to all observations.

This problem is commonly addressed by use of a two-part model (3, 25, 30) in which the first part predicts the probability that the patient had nonzero or zero cost and the second part predicts the level of cost conditional upon having positive cost. The first part is generally fitted by use of a logistic or probit model to the dichotomous variable defined by whether the patient had nonzero costs or not. The second part is fitted by use of the standard models discussed above, such as GLM, to predict cost in the subset of patients whose cost is positive. Expected cost for individual patients is then derived by multiplying the predictions from the two components together. Two-part models exploit the mixed distribution of cost data and also allow evaluation of whether the treatment lowers cost by affecting the probability of an individual having a cost incurring event alone, the level of cost incurred given that there was a cost incurring event, or both.

5.5. Summary and recommendations

Because cost-effectiveness (and cost-benefit) analysis should be based on differences in the arithmetic means, we should report these means and their difference, measures of variability and precision, and an indication of whether or not the observed differences in the arithmetic mean are likely to have occurred by chance. Reporting medians and other percentiles of the distribution is also useful in describing cost.

Evaluation of the difference in arithmetic mean cost and determination of the likelihood that it is due to chance is complicated by the fact that health care cost is typically characterized by highly skewed distributions with long and sometimes awkwardly heavy right tails. The existence of such distributions has led some observers to reject the use of arithmetic means and the common statistical methods used for their analysis, such as *t* tests of untransformed cost. Given that statistical inference about statistics other than the arithmetic mean need not be representative of inference about the arithmetic mean, use of these alternative statistics divorces inference from estimation.

Given the multiple problems confronting analysis of cost, it is optimal to perform both univariate and multivariable analysis of difference in the arithmetic mean of cost. However, common characteristics of the distribution of cost can cause problems for a large number of the available multivariable techniques. It is most likely the case that no single model will always be most appropriate for estimating cost differences associated with medical therapies. While Manning and Mullahy (2001) have proposed methods for selecting an appropriate multivariable model, in practice, the small sample sizes and dramatically skewed distributions of cost in clinical trials may make such selection of the optimal model difficult, if not impossible. Thus investigators should consider estimating and reporting a number of different models, thus providing readers with a measure of the degree of variation in the estimates that is due to model uncertainty – the conceptual equivalent of using sensitivity analysis to determine the robustness of numerical analyses.

References

1. Hosmer Jr. DW, Lemeshow S. *Applied Survival Analysis*. New York: John Wiley & Sons, Inc., 1999.
2. Hosmer Jr. DW, Lemeshow S. *Applied Logistic Regression*, 2nd ed. New York: John Wiley & Sons, Inc., 2000.
3. Duan N. Smearing estimate: a nonparametric retransformation method. *J Am Stat Assoc*. 1983; 78: 605–10.
4. Thompson SG, Barber JA. How should cost data in pragmatic randomised trials be analysed? *BMJ*. 2000; 320: 1197–200.
5. Ramsey S, Willke R, Briggs A, Brown R, Buxton M, Chawla A, Cook J, Glick H, Liljas B, Petitti D, Reed S. Best practices for economic analysis alongside clinical trials: an ISPOR RCT-CEA Task Force report. *Value Health* 2005; 8: 521–33.
6. Hurley J. An overview of normative economics of the health sector, Chapter 2. In *Handbook of Health Economics*, Volume 1A, edited by A.J. Culyer and J.P. Newhouse. Amsterdam: Elsevier Science B.V., 2000, p. 61.
7. Gayan AK. Significance of difference between the means of two non-normal samples. *Biometrika* 1950; 37: 399–408.
8. Pearson ES, Please NW. Relation between the shape of population distribution and the robustness of four simple test statistics. *Biometrika* 1975; 62: 223–41.
9. Geary RC. Testing for normality. *Biometrika* 1947; 36: 353–69.

10. **Doshi JA, Glick HA, Polsky DP.** Analyses of cost data in economic evaluations conducted alongside randomized controlled trials. *Value Health* 2006; 9: 334–40.

11. **Mann HB, Whitney DR.** On a test of whether one of 2 random variables is stochastically larger than the other. *Ann Math Stat.* 1947; 18: 50–60.

12. **Wilcoxon F.** Individual comparisons by ranking methods. *Biomet Bull.* 1945; 1: 80–3.

13. **Conover WJ.** *Practical Nonparametric Statistics*, 3rd ed. New York: John Wiley & Sons, 1999.

14. **Kruskal WH, Wallis WA.** Use of ranks in one-criterion variance analysis. *J Am Stat Assoc.* 1952; 47: 583–621.

15. **Manning WG.** The logged dependent variable, heteroscedasticity, and the retransformation problem. *J Health Econ.* 1998; 17(3): 283–95.

16. **Barber JA, Thompson SG.** Analysis of cost data in randomized trials: an application of the non-parametric bootstrap. *Stat Med.* 2000; 19: 3219–36.

17. **Efron B, Tibshirani RJ.** *An Introduction to the Bootstrap.* New York: Chapman and Hall, 1993.

18. **Davison AC, Hinkley DV.** *Bootstrap Methods and their Application.* Cambridge: Cambridge University Press, 1997.

19. **Sokal RR, Rohlf FJ.** Biometry: *The Principles and Practice of Statistics in Biological Research.* London: W.H. Freeman & Company, 1995.

20. **O'Hagan A, Stevens JW.** Assessing and comparing costs: how robust are the bootstrap and methods based on asymptotic normality? *Health Econ.* 2003; 12: 33–49.

21. **Kennedy P.** A Guide to Econometrics, 5th ed. Cambridge, MA: MIT Press, 2003.

22. **Manning WG, Mullahy J.** Estimating log models: to transform or not to transform? *J Health Econ.* 2001; 20: 461–94.

23. **Nelder JA, Wedderburn RWM.** Generalized linear models. *J Roy Stat Soc A.* 1972; 135: 370–84.

24. **McCullagh P, Nelder JA.** *Generalized Linear Models*, 2nd ed. London: Chapman & Hall, 1989.

25. **Blough DK, Madden CW, Hornbrook MC.** Modeling risk using generalized linear models. *J Health Econ.* 1999; 18: 153–71.

26. **Pregibon D.** Goodness of link tests for generalized linear models. *Appl Stat.* 1980; 29: 15–24.

27. **Copas JB.** Regression, prediction and shrinkage (with discussion). *J Roy Stat Soc B.* 1983; 45: 311–54.

28. **Basu A, Rathouz PJ.** Estimating marginal and incremental effects on health outcomes using flexible link and variance function models. *Biostat.* 2005; 6: 93–109.

29. **Manning WG, Basu A, Mullahy J.** Generalized modeling approaches to risk adjustment of skewed outcomes data. National Bureau of Economic Research, Technical Working Paper 293. http://www.nber.org/papers/T0293

30. **Lipscomb J, Ancukiewicz M, Parmigiani G, Hasselblad V, Samsa G, Matchar DB.** Predicting the cost of illness: a comparison of alternative models applied to stroke. *Med Decis Making* 1998; 15(suppl): S39–56.

Chapter 6

Analyzing censored cost

Incomplete data are inevitable in economic analyses conducted alongside trials. Cost – and effect – data may be incomplete due to item-level missingness; for example, data for visit 3 might be missing, but data for visits 1 and 2 and data for all visits after 3 are available. In what follows, we refer to such data as missing. Cost data may also be incomplete because of loss to follow-up; for example, data for visits 1 and 2 might be available, but all data after visit 2 are missing. We call these data censored.

Our primary focus in this chapter is on censored cost data rather than on missing data. The problem of missing data is not new and the biostatistical literature has given substantial attention to appropriate methods for handling these data. Imputation methods for missing data have been extensively studied and the multiple imputation approach has been widely recommended by most experts, given that it reflects the uncertainty that is inherent when replacing missing data [1]. On the other hand, there has been more recent statistical interest in addressing censored cost data which has led to the proposal of several methods of estimation that explicitly account for censoring in a health-economic context.

In this chapter, we discuss the different mechanisms of censoring, review three tests for diagnosing the mechanism of censoring, and briefly describe eight approaches for addressing censored cost data. As we noted in Chapter 5, while our focus here is on the analysis of cost, many of the same techniques can also be used to analyze effect.

6.1. The problem

Censored cost data often occur in randomized trials that follow participants for clinically meaningful lengths of time. Failure to address this censoring can lead to inconsistent estimates of arithmetic mean cost [2], and thus efforts should be made to overcome the problems it poses.

Data on cost, medical service use, or effect are considered censored if their collection ends before the study's period of observation is complete. One can think of censored cost data in the same way as one thinks of censoring in survival analysis. An observation on a variable is right censored if all you know about the variable is that it is greater than some value.

In survival analysis, the censored variable is typically the time of occurrence for some event, and right censoring is common. Cases are right censored because observation is terminated before the event occurs. For example, if the censored variable is the time from randomization until death (in years), you may know only that the variable is greater than 5 years, in which case the person's death time is right censored at 5 years.

In cost analysis, the censored variable is typically the sum of a flow of cost, and cases are right censored because observation is terminated before the flow ends. For example, if the censored variable is cost after randomization until death, you may know only that the cost is greater than 20,000, in which case the person's cost is right censored at 20,000. While right censoring is still the norm, participants can "drop in" to the cost study, in the sense that we may observe a participant's cost from visit 4 until the end of the trial, but not observe cost for the first three visits. In this case, the cost data are left censored.

In some clinical trials, censoring of cost may arise because the trial randomizes participants over time, but ends follow-up on a fixed calendar date, for example, when a certain number of outcomes are reached. In other cases, censored cost data arise due to patient attrition from study or participants being lost to follow-up. Such censoring generally follows a monotonic pattern. Of note, in this context death does not represent censoring of cost or effect data. It represents complete data in that no further cost nor effect is accrued.

To appropriately account for the effect of such censoring, one must understand the reason the data are censored, which we refer to as the the mechanism of censoring.

6.2. **Mechanisms of censoring**

Many mechanisms can generate censoring of cost data. For example, a participant may be impossible to locate during the follow-up period; he or she may drop out of the study for reasons related or unrelated to the treatment under study; in some – inappropriate – trial designs, the occurrence of a clinical outcome, such as the failure of the study therapy, may exclude a participant from further follow-up; or the study may enroll participants over a period of months or years and discontinue follow-up on a fixed calendar date. This last mechanism represents a form of administrative censoring that we refer to as rolling admission with a fixed stopping date.

Most censoring mechanisms can be classified into one of three categories: missing completely at random (MCAR), missing at random (MAR), and missing not at random (MNAR) which is also referred to as nonignorably missing [3]. The first occurs when the reason for the censored cost data is independent of the mechanism that generates cost. It implies that the cost for participants who have incomplete follow-up is the same, except for random variation, as the cost for participants with complete data. As an example, the censoring that occurs because of rolling admission and a fixed stopping data is usually considered MCAR, because the end of follow-up is unrelated to what is happening to the patient.

MAR censoring occurs when censored cost data are correlated in an observable way with the mechanism that generates cost. That is, after adjustment for the observable differences between the complete and censored cases, the cost for participants who have incomplete follow-up is the same, except for random variation, as that for participants with complete data. For example, men in a study may be more difficult to locate during follow-up than women, but if sex is controlled for, participants with censored data may have the same cost as those without censored data.

MNAR or nonignorably missing censoring occurs when the mechanism that generates the censored observations is correlated with the mechanism that generates cost. In other words, the cost of participants who are censored differs in unpredictable ways from the cost of those without censored data. Hence, the censoring cannot be ignored. The censoring that occurs when participants discontinue both the therapy under study and study follow-up after a serious adverse event may be considered MNAR.

6.3. Diagnosing the mechanism of censoring

No direct tests of the mechanism of censoring are available, because given the data are censored, one cannot compare the data that are unavailable to those that are. However, sufficient, although not necessary, indirect tests exist for ruling out MCAR versus either MAR or MNAR and for distinguishing MAR from MNAR.

6.3.1. Ruling out MCAR

We can rule out an MCAR mechanism if clinical and demographic characteristics of participants with censored data differ significantly from the characteristics of participants without censored data. For example, Table 6.1 shows such a comparison from a clinical trial evaluating a therapy for AIDS. Significant differences were observed between those with and without censored data for: the CD4 count before randomization, the percentage of patients either hospitalized or who used the emergency department before

Table 6.1 Comparison of clinical characteristics of participants with complete versus censored cost data

Variable	Therapy 1			Therapy 2		
	Complete cases	Censored cases	p value	Complete cases	Censored cases	p value
Sample size	131	169	–	138	158	–
CD4 count before randomization, cells/mm^3	169	119	0.0001	181	105	0.0001
Hospitalized during 6 months before randomization, %	16.0	26.6	0.03	14.5	30.2	0.001
Used emergency department during 3 months before randomization, %	5.3	9.5	0.18	2.9	8.8	0.03
Met European AIDS criteria,%	28.2	43.2	0.008	21.0	47.2	0.0001
Met European criteria for AIDS-related complex, %	76.3	67.5	0.09	84.8	65.4	0.0001
Number of current AIDS-defining conditions	0.95	1.1	0.30	0.67	1.1	0.0001

randomization, and the percentage who met European criteria for AIDS or AIDS-defining complex. Note that we make treatment-specific comparisons of the characteristics of those with and without censored data, because the mechanism of censoring can differ between treatment groups. These results provide evidence that the censoring mechanism is not MCAR.

We can also rule out MCAR if – during the periods prior to censoring – the cost for participants who eventually have censored data differs significantly from the cost for those who never have censored data during the same periods. Table 6.2 shows a comparison of cost stratified by treatment group, month, and whether or not the participant ever had censored cost data during the first year of follow-up. Note that we do not report results for the 12th month, because no participants with censored data had cost data in this month. The row averages at the bottom of the table indicate that participants who received therapy 1 and ever had any censored cost data had a monthly

Table 6.2 Comparison of costs among participants who eventually have censored cost data versus those who never have censored cost data

Month	Therapy 1*						Therapy 2*					
	Complete cases			Censored cases			Complete cases			Censored cases		
	Mean	SD	N	Mean	SD	N	Mean	SD	N	Mean	SD	N
1	528	459	131	897	1642	169	216	472	138	590	1178	158
2	523	448	131	503	553	145	303	1493	138	510	952	152
3	518	468	131	740	1292	117	217	427	138	547	1209	141
4	522	512	131	773	1762	99	226	580	138	360	937	126
5	543	484	131	880	2217	87	219	363	138	637	1977	114
6	548	531	131	457	447	69	296	803	138	687	1948	102
7	531	466	131	1120	4630	56	464	1505	138	447	1044	84
8	464	363	131	753	1119	50	230	483	138	1199	4449	67
9	499	390	131	738	2088	41	391	1294	138	678	2167	52
10	485	376	131	564	1447	22	365	1194	138	566	1816	33
11	490	407	131	131	94	9	212	347	138	1019	2139	11
Average	514	448	1441	741	1840	864	285	928	1518	595	1787	1040

*$p < 0.001$ that the average costs among participants who ever have censored data are greater than the average costs among participants who never have censored cost data.

cost that on average was 227 (741–514) greater than participant who never had any censored data ($p < 0.001$). Participants who received therapy 2 and ever had any censored cost data had a monthly cost that on average was 310 (595–285) greater than participants those who never had any censored data ($p < 0.001$). We estimated the reported p-values by use of a generalized linear model with a gamma family (chosen by use of the modified Park test [see p. **108, 109**, Chapter 5]) and a log link to predict cost per interval as a function of whether the participant was ever censored, controlling for month of follow-up. In doing so, we estimated robust standard errors and accounted for the multiple observations that were available for participants. These results provide additional evidence against the MCAR assumption.

6.3.2. **Ruling out MAR**

Finally, we can rule out an MAR mechanism if, after controlling for the probability of being censored, the cost for participants who eventually have censored data differs significantly from the cost for those who never have censored data. In such instances, the data are said to be MNAR.

As we indicate below, determination of mechanism can affect the analytic technique that is appropriate for addressing censored data. For example, methods that are appropriate for addressing data that are censored via an MCAR mechanism may not be appropriate for data that are censored via an MAR or MNAR mechanism. On the other hand, if the mechanism is MCAR, one may not need to incur the cost of methods that are appropriate for data that are censored via an MNAR mechanism. At the same time, lack of evidence to reject one of these mechanisms differs from the existence of evidence that is indicative of the actual mechanism. Thus, we may want to adopt methods that protect against misdiagnosis of the mechanism.

6.4. **Addressing censored cost data**

In what follows, we briefly review eight methods (several of which have two variants) for addressing censored cost data. The best methods use all available information; yield unbiased estimates of arithmetic mean cost, and thus of the difference in this cost; and are efficient.

6.4.1. **Naive methods**

There are two commonly used naive approaches for addressing censored data. In the first, often referred to as complete case analysis, observations with any censored data are excluded from analysis. Complete case analysis is problematic in that it yields results that are biased toward the cost of the patients with shorter survival times. It does so because patients with longer survival times are more likely to be censored [4,5]. This type of analysis has further limitations in that it discards data from patients with censored cost data, which leads to a loss of both information and statistical power.

The second naive method, often referred to as full sample analysis, includes data from all participants but acts as though the observed data represents complete observations. Full sample analysis is problematic in that it always yields estimates of individual treatment group means that are downward biased [5]. While we know the direction of the bias for the individual group means, we cannot, however, be sure of the direction of the bias for the difference in means, because differential downward bias of each group's mean can lead to a predicted difference that is greater than or less than the actual difference.

A third approach, which while not naive is also mistaken, is to apply survival analysis techniques to the problem of cost estimation by treating cost as a potentially right censored survival time and attaching a censoring indicator to observed total cost [6–10]. This strategy has been shown to be invalid [4,11,12] because – unlike time – participants usually do not accumulate cost with a common rate function. In general, participants who accumulate cost at higher rates will have a higher cumulative cost at both the censoring time and the survival time than will participants with lower accumulation rates. Given this positive correlation, the assumption underlying the validity of these approaches – independence between the variable of interest (cost at event) and its censoring variable (cost at censoring) – is generally violated with cost data.

6.4.2. **Lin 1997 method**

Lin and colleagues [4] proposed an interval method to analyze censored medical cost data when detailed patient cost histories are available. In this method, we first divide the study period into a number of smaller time intervals, for example months or quarters. Second, we calculate the probability that study participants survive to the beginning of each interval, for example at the beginning of the month or quarter, by use of the Kaplan–Meier method. Third, we calculate the mean cost per interval among those alive and available for follow-up during the interval. Fourth, we weight the mean cost per interval by the probability of survival to the interval. This weighting yields an estimate of mean cost during each interval that accounts for dropout and death. Finally, we sum the weighted cost estimates for each of the intervals to obtain an estimate of mean total cost for the study period.

In this same article, Lin and colleagues [4] proposed a second approach that is appropriate when interval-specific data are not available.

The Lin 1997 method is appropriate for data that are censored by means of an MCAR mechanism because it assumes that participants who are lost to follow-up have the same survival and cost as participants who are available for follow-up at the time of dropout. Conceptually, the Lin 1997 method is similar to an imputation based on average cost per period, but it includes added information about the survival of censored subjects.

6.4.3. **Bang and Tsiatis method**

Similar to the Lin 1997 method, the Bang and Tsiatis method [13] has one variant that is appropriate when interval-specific cost data are available and another that is appropriate when total cost is all that is available. When interval-specific cost data are available, we again first partition the study period into a number of smaller time intervals. Second, we derive estimates of cost incurred in each interval by weighting the interval-specific cost for uncensored patients by the inverse probability of their being observed in the interval (i.e., not being censored). The probability of being observed in the interval is derived by use of a Kaplan–Meier estimator, but as Young [14] has indicated, in this case the estimator is based on the prediction of censoring, not the prediction of death (i.e., the failure indicator is coded as a 1 for observations that are censored and is coded as a 0 for those who die). This estimator differs from more commonly reported Kaplan–Meier estimators in that in most epidemiologic studies, they are used to predict death or a nonfatal outcome such as myocardial infraction (death or infraction are coded as a 1, censoring is coded as a 0). Third, we derive the estimate of mean total cost by summing over these intervals and dividing by the overall sample size, including both uncensored and censored observations.

The intuition behind accounting for censoring by weighting cost by the inverse probability of being observed is that these weights are greatest for those who are expected to be censored but for whom data are available. We weight these observations more heavily because participants who are like these observations generally have been censored during follow-up and their cost data is not available for us to include in our estimate. Weights are smallest for those who are expected to be uncensored and for whom data are available. We weight them less heavily, because participants who are like them generally are not censored, and thus we already are including most of their cost data in our estimate. As Lin has noted [15], weighting by the inverse of the probability of being observed has a long history, beginning with Horvitz and Thompson in 1952 [16], being introduced into the analysis of censored survival data by Koul *et al.* [17], and being introduced into the analysis of quality adjusted survival time by Zhao and Tsiatis [18].

In the second variant, when interval-specific cost data are unavailable, total study cost from the uncensored patients – those who died during the trial and those with complete cost information for the trial period – is weighted by the inverse probability of being observed. As with the first method, this probability is calculated by use of the Kaplan–Meier censoring probability estimator. The resulting weighted cost estimates are then summed and divided by the overall sample size to obtain the mean total cost estimate in the presence of censoring.

As with the Lin 1997 method, the Bang and Tsiatis method is appropriate for data that are censored by means of an MCAR mechanism.

6.4.4. Carides regression method

The Carides regression method [19] is a parametric method based on the assumption that patients' total study cost can be modeled as a function of survival time. This method consists of two steps. First, a regression model that best fits the data is used to predict total cost as a function of survival time. This model is estimated using cost data from uncensored patients only – i.e., those with complete study cost or those who died during the study – to avoid bias in the regression estimates due to censoring. Like the other interval-based non-parametric methods discussed above, the study period is divided into smaller time intervals. Second, the mean expected cost for those patients who die within each interval is calculated and weighted by the Kaplan–Meier probability of death in that particular interval. The estimate of the mean total study cost is obtained by summing over the weighted estimates across all intervals.

The Carides regression method may be appropriate for data that are censored by means of an MAR mechanism.

6.4.5. Lin 2000 method

In 2000, Lin [15] proposed a method that, unlike his 1997 method, uses weighted ordinary least squares (OLS) regression models to predict cost while controlling for patient and clinical covariates. As with the Lin 1997 and Bang and Tsiatis methods, the Lin 2000 method can be used to calculate cost subdivided by interval or total cost. Focusing on the interval-specific method, participants contribute data during the intervals in which they are observed (i.e., until the period in which they are censored). The regression results are adjusted for censoring by weighting the observations by the inverse of the probability of an individual being observed in the interval. The probability weights are obtained from either Kaplan–Meier or other survival analysis models such as Cox regressions, for which – like the Bang and Tsiatis weights – censoring is coded as a 1 and death is coded as a 0. The resulting weighted regression coefficients are then applied to all patients in the sample (i.e., both uncensored and censored) to obtain a predicted cost per patient, which in turn is used to calculate mean total cost.

The Lin 2000 method is appropriate for data that are censored by means of an MAR mechanism because it controls for a series of covariates that may be related to censoring.

There have been a number of authors who have extended the Lin 2000 method. For example, Jain and Strawderman [20] did so by incorporating inverse probability weighting in a hazard regression model for the distribution of lifetime costs. Willan *et al.* [21] extended Lin's method to the comparison of cost and effect in two treatments groups in a longitudinal framework by use of seemingly unrelated regression equations. Baser *et al.* [22] extend Lin's methods by allowing incorporation of time-dependent covariates using a panel data model.

Finally, Lin himself extended the model in 2003 [23]. Because of the problems that face the use OLS regression to predict cost, he modified the model so that it could be used with generalized linear models (see our discussion in Chapter 5). These models provide a flexible means of assessing the effects of covariates on cost accumulation.

6.4.6. Multiple imputation methods

As we indicated at the beginning of this chapter, multiple imputation has routinely been used to address problems posed by missing data [24,25]. More recently, it has been employed in clinical trial-based analyses to address problems posed by censored data [26–28].

In a number of these methods, e.g., Lavori [26] and Oostenbrink [27], a propensity score, representing the probability of being censored, is used to stratify participants into quintiles of risk for censoring. In repeated datasets, one randomly draws data from uncensored observations in the same quintile of risk to "fill in" the censored data. Each of the resulting datasets is thus "complete" and can be analyzed by use of the methods we described in Chapter 5 without concern for censoring. The final point estimate is derived from the means in the repeated samples. The standard errors account for both within- and between-sample variation. Oostenbrink and Al [28], on the other hand, used regression based methods, wherein a regression is estimated for each censored value conditional upon covariates at baseline or lagged time periods.

6.5. Comparison of different methods

Several recent articles have compared a number of these different methods for addressing censored cost data [2,5,14]. All three articles document that use of naive methods to estimate average cost can lead to bias in the presence of censoring. Young [14] also provides a demonstration that the use of method 3 above, which attaches a censoring variable to observed total cost, also leads to biased estimates of the mean.

Raikou and McGuire [5] assessed the empirical performance of the Lin 1997 and Bang and Tsiatis methods with and without interval-specific cost data. The estimators were compared in terms of bias and efficiency under extreme conditions by use of observed and simulated datasets all of which exhibited heavy censoring. They found that both the Lin 1997 and the Bang and Tsiatis methods performed well under all conditions. Given that both methods require the same amount of cost information, Raikou and McGuire suggest that the Bang and Tsiatis method might be preferred because it is not restricted by the pattern of the censoring distribution and is therefore more general than the Lin 1997 method. More recently, these authors [29] have reported that the Lin 2000 method performs as well as the Lin 1997 and Bang and Tsiatis methods.

Young [14] compared 7 of the 8 methods we have outlined (she did not compare the multiple imputation methods). If one is solely interested in the point estimate of mean total cost, she found that the Lin 1997 method without interval cost data and Carides regression method performed best. Neither method, however, did well at predicting standard errors. When both point estimates and standard errors are of interest, Young reports that the Bang and Tsiatis method using interval-specific cost data was consistently the most accurate method.

6.6. **How much censored data is too much?**

No clear guidance exists for how much censoring is too much. One hears of rules of thumb that suggest that if 5–10% of the total data are censored, then adjusting for this censoring will have too little an impact on the study result to make the adjustment exercise worthwhile. While our own experience supports this suggestion, we have been unable to track down either these rules of thumb or the evidence that might support them. Possibly because it was difficult to provide citations for such rules of thumb, the ISPOR RCT-CEA task-force recommended that, "ignoring small amounts of missing data is acceptable if a reasonable case can be made that doing so is unlikely to bias treatment group comparisons" [1]. The authors did not provide guidance as to what form such evidence might take.

We should note that any recommendations about whether we need to account for censored data are based on the amount of data that are censored, not upon the proportion of participants who have censored data. Table 6.3 uses the data from Table 6.2 in a worked example to illustrate this difference (see Box 6.1). A total of 596 participants initiated follow-up in the trial. By the end of 12 months, 327 participants (55%) had been censored. The potential number of periods of observation was 7152. Those who were never censored contributed data for 3228 periods; those who were ever censored contributed data for 1904; and the total number of periods with censored data were 2020 (7152–5132), or 28%. Of course, by any criteria that is too much censoring to ignore.

Table 6.3 Summary of censored data

Variable	Never censored	Ever censored	Total
Participants, N			
Therapy 1	131	169	300
Therapy 2	138	158	296
Total	269	327	596
Participants, %			
Therapy 1	44	56	100
Therapy 2	47	53	100
Total	45	55	100
Periods with data available, N			
Therapy 1	1572	864[†]	2436
Therapy 2	1656	1040[‡]	2696
Total	3228	1904	5132
Potential periods of observation, N*			
Therapy 1	1572	2028	3600
Therapy 2	1656	1896	3552
Total	3228	3924	7152
Periods with data available, %			
Therapy 1	100	43	68
Therapy 2	100	55	76
Total	100	49	72
Periods with censored data, %	0	51	28

*Number of participants × 12. Death is not considered a censoring event, and periods after death are counted as observations with known outcome.

[†]Column 7 total, Table 6.2.

[‡]Column 13 total, Table 6.2.

Box 6.1 Calculating the proportion of the data that are missing

Step 1. For each treatment group and for the overall trial, sum the total number of participants who never and ever have censored data. As seen in Table 6.3, 131 participants who received therapy 1 never had any censored data, 169 who received this therapy ever had any censored data; 138 participants who received therapy 2 never had any censored data, 158 who received this therapy did.

Step 2. Divide the numbers of participants with and without any censored data in each treatment group and the trial as a whole by the total number of participants within the same groups. As shown in Table 6.3, the results of these calculations indicate that 56% of participants in who received therapy 1 had any censored data, 53% who received therapy 2 had any censored data, and 55% of all participants in the trial had any censored data.

Step 3. Sum the monthly number of observations for participants who received therapy 1 and therapy 2 and who did and did not ever have censored data. For those who ever had censored data, the correct numbers come from the column totals for columns 7 and 13 in Table 6.2. For those who never had censored data, we must remember to add 131 and 138 to the column totals for those who received therapy 1 and 2, respectively, because these participants also contributed complete data for the 12th month of follow-up (note that no one who was censored contributed data for this month). The results of these calculations are shown in Table 6.3.

Step 4. Calculate the total number potential periods of observation. Because we treat periods after death as if the values for the month are known (0), for those who were never censored, we multiply the number of participants by 12. Because we do not know survival status after censoring, for those who were ever censored, we also multiply the number of these participants by 12.

Step 5. Divide the number of observations by the number of potential observations. As seen in Table 6.3, those who never had censored data contributed 100% of their observations. Participants with any censored data contributed 43, 55, and 49% of their observations for therapy 1, 2, and both therapies, respectively. When we combine the 0% censoring among 45% of the participants with no censoring and the 51% censoring among 55% of the participants with any censoring, we find that 28% of the total observations were censored.

6.7. **Interval-specific analysis**

As we have indicated, a common feature of approaches for addressing censored data is to divide total cost into a set of interval-specific cost estimates, and to use all data from participants until the interval when their data are censored. In addition to enabling the use of all available data, this approach has other advantages that recommend its adoption even when we are not addressing problems of censored data. For example, if the illness episode extends beyond the period of follow-up in the trial, i.e., if we are evaluating a therapy for a chronic condition, this approach allows us to observe time trends in the data. As shown in Fig. 6.1, the fact that a therapy saved $720 over 4 years does not mean that it necessarily will continue to save money after follow-up is discontinued. In this case, the bulk of the savings were observed during the first year of the trial. Thereafter, there was little or no saving.

These interval-specific analyses represent a form of repeated measures analysis, in that the same participant contributes multiple observations to the data. In general, these multiple observations for the same participant will be correlated. We should account for this correlation in our analysis, otherwise the resulting standard errors will too small.

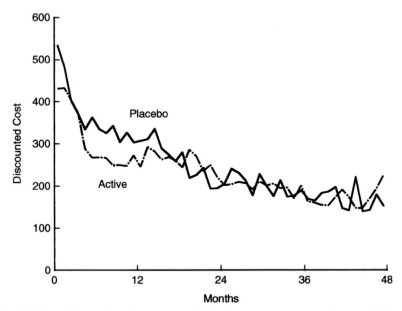

Fig. 6.1 Monthly cost data for active and placebo treatment groups Source: Glick *et al.* [30]

Reproduced from Glick H, Cook J, Kinosian B, Pitt B, Bourassa MG, Pouleur H, Gerth W 'Costs and Effects of Enalapril Therapy in Patients with Symptomatic Heart Failure: An Economic Analysis of the Studies of Left Ventricular Dysfunction (SOLVD) Treatment Trial' *Journal of Cardiac Failure* 1995; 1: 371–80 with permission from Elsevier.

6.8. **Discussion**

Censored data are common in trials, and they are often not addressed in the analysis. For example, in their review of 115 economic assessments based on patient-level data from clinical trials that were published in 2003, Doshi and colleagues [31] found that 26 studies (23%) reported no attrition, 67 (58%) reported some incomplete cost data, and the remaining 22 (19%) did not indicate whether or not complete follow-up was achieved. Among the 67 studies that reported some incomplete cost data, none reported tests of the censoring mechanism and only 19 (28%) made some attempt to address the incompleteness of the data, usually by some form of imputation. Only two of the 67 studies used a statistical approach like the ones described in this chapter.

When cost data are incomplete, the amount of incomplete data and the statistical method adopted to address the problems posed by incomplete data should routinely be reported in trial-based analyses [1]. Ideally, one should also report the results of tests for diagnosing the censoring mechanism. When there is a substantial amount of censored data, ignoring it or using one of the naive methods for addressing it will lead to biased results. While new methods continue to be introduced, as O'Hagan and Stevens [2] have recommended, the Lin 1997 or Bang and Tsiatis methods are reasonable [minimum] approaches for addressing this censoring.

Understanding the censoring mechanism allows us to determine whether we need a method that is appropriate for data that have MCAR or MAR censoring mechanisms. We have proposed indirect tests of mechanism, but determination of the mechanism is aided by the collection of as much information as possible about the reasons for drop-out. One should also consider what the likely course of a participant is once she stops taking study medications: is all benefit lost, or will she switch to an alternative therapy that will provide equal protection? In addition, if the censoring mechanism cannot be well diagnosed, analyses should be conducted to assess the sensitivity of results to plausible alternative specifications of the mechanism.

While in this chapter we focused on methods for addressing censored data once it has occurred, avoiding such data in the first place is the best method for addressing censored cost. As we indicated in Chapter 2, concerted efforts should be taken during the design of the trial and while the data are being collected to avoid both censored and missing data. In addition, because some censoring is inevitable, attempts should be made to identify and collect information on covariates that are useful for predicting this censoring. Moreover, as O'Hagan and Stevens [2] have recommended, because interval data yield greater statistical efficiency than do data on total cost, patient cost should always be recorded in such a way that it can be subdivided into intervals.

Finally, all of the methods we have reviewed address data whose censoring mechanism is either MCAR or MAR. Unfortunately, when there is evidence of an MNAR censoring mechanism, the literature provides substantially less systematic advice about how the censoring problem should be addressed. As the ISPOR RCT-CEA taskforce noted, when nonrandom censoring occurs, "external data sources for similar patients may be required to both identify and address it" [1].

References

1. Ramsey S, Willke R, Briggs A, Brown R, Buxton M, Chawla A, Cook J, Glick H, Liljas B, Petitti D, Reed S. Best practices for economic analysis alongside clinical trials: an ISPOR RCT-CEA Task Force report. *Value Health*. 2005; 8: 521–33.

2. O'Hagan A, Stevens JW. On estimators of medical costs with censored data. *J Health Econ*. 2004; 23: 615–25.

3. Rubin DB. Inference and missing data. *Biometrika* 1976; 63: 581–92.

4. Lin DY, Feuer EJ, Etzioni R, Wax Y. Estimating medical costs from incomplete follow-up data. *Biometrics* 1997; 53: 113–28.

5. Raikou M, McGuire A. Estimating medical care costs under conditions of censoring. *J Health Econ*. 2004; 23: 443–70.

6. Quesenberry CP. A survival analysis of hospitalizations among patients with acquired immunodeficiency syndrome. *Am J Public Health* 1989; 79: 1643–7.

7. Hiatt RA, Quesenberry Jr. CP, Selby JV, Fireman BH, Knight A. The cost of acquired immunodeficiency syndrome in Northern California: the experience of a large prepaid health plan. *Arch Intern Med*. 1990; 150: 833–8.

8. Dudley RA, Harrell FE, Smith LR, Mark DB, Califf RM, Pryor DB, Glower D, Lipscomb J, Hlatky M. Comparison of analytic models for estimating the effect of clinical factors on the cost of coronary artery bypass graft surgery. *J Clin Epidemiol*. 1993; 46: 261–71.

9. Fenn P, McGuire A, Phillips V, Backhouse M, Jones D. The analysis of censored treatment cost data in economic evaluation. *Med Care* 1995; 22: 851–63.

10. Harrell F, Lee K, Mark D. Multivariable prognostic models: issues in developing models, evaluating assumptions and adequacy, and measuring and reducing errors. *Stat Med*. 1996; 15: 361–87.

11. Hallstrom AP, Sullivan SD. On estimating costs of economic evaluation in failure time studies. *Med Care* 1998; 36: 433–6.

12. Lipscomb J, Ancukiewicz M, Parmigiani G, Hasselblad V, Samsa G, Matchar DBJ. Predicting the cost of illness: a comparison of alternative models applied to stroke. *Med Decis Making* 1998; 18: S39–56.

13. Bang H, Tsiatis AA. Estimating medical costs with censored data. *Biometrika* 2000; 87: 329–43.

14. Young T. Estimating mean total costs in the presence of censoring, a comparative assessment of methods. *Pharmacoeconomics* 2005; 23(12) 1229–40.

15. **Lin DY.** Linear regression analysis of censored medical costs. *Biostatistics* 2000; 1: 35–47.

16. **Horvitz DG, Thompson DJ.** A generalization of sampling without replacement from a finite universe. *JASA.* 1952; 47: 663–85.

17. **Koul H, Susarla V, Van Ryzin J.** Regression analysis with randomly right-censored data. *Ann Stat* 1981; 9: 1276–88.

18. **Zhao H, Tsiatis AA.** A consistent estimator for the distribution of quality-adjusted survival time. *Biometrika* 1997; 84: 339–48.

19. **Carides GW, Heyse JF, Iglewicz B.** A regression-based method for estimating mean treatment cost in the presence of right-censoring. *Biostatistics* 2000; 1: 299–313.

20. **Jain AR, Strawderman RL.** Flexible hazard regression modeling for medical cost data. *Biostatistics* 2002; 3: 101–18.

21. **Willan AR, Lin DY, Manca A.** Regression methods for cost-effectiveness analysis with censored data. *Stat Med.* 2005; 24: 131–45.

22. **Baser O, Gardiner JC, Bradley CJ, Yuce H, Given C.** Longitudinal analysis of censored medical cost data. *Health Econ.* 2006; 15: 513–25.

23. **Lin DY.** Regression analysis of incomplete medical cost data. *Stat Med.* 2003; 22: 1181–200.

24. **Rubin DB.** *Multiple imputations in sample surveys – a phenomenological Bayesian approach.* ASA Proceedings of the Section on Research Methods, Alexandria, Virginia: American Statistical Association, 1978, 20–28.

25. **Rubin DB.** *Multiple Imputation for Nonresponse in Surveys.* New York: John Wiley, 1978.

26. **Lavori PW, Dawson R, Shera D.** A multiple imputation strategy for clinical trials with truncation of patient data. *Stat Med.* 1995; 14: 1913–25.

27. **Oostenbrink JB, Al MJ, Rutten-van Molken MPMH.** Methods to analyse cost data of patients who withdraw in a clinical trial setting. *Pharmacoeconomics* 2003; 21: 1103–12.

28. **Oostenbrink JB, Al MJ.** The analysis of incomplete cost data due to dropout. *Health Econ.* 2005; 14: 763–76.

29. **Raikou M, McGuire A.** Estimating costs for economic evaluation, Chapter 40. In *The Elgar Companion to Health Economics*, edited by A.M. Jones. Cheltenham, UK: Edward Elgar, 2006.

30. **Glick H, Cook J, Kinosian B, Pitt B, Bourassa MG, Pouleur H, Gerth W.** Costs and Effects of Enalapril Therapy in Patients with Symptomatic Heart Failure: An Economic Analysis of the Studies of Left Ventricular Dysfunction (SOLVD) Treatment Trial. *J Card Fail.* 1995; 1: 371–80.

31. **Doshi JA, Glick HA, Polsky DP.** Analyses of cost data in economic evaluations conducted alongside randomized controlled trials. *Value Health* 2006; 9: 334–40.

Chapter 7

Comparing cost and effect: point estimates for cost-effectiveness ratios and net monetary benefit

Once we have estimated the difference in cost and effect, we need to jointly assess these two outcomes to determine whether the data support the value for the cost of one of the therapies under evaluation. In this chapter, we describe two methods for developing point estimates for the difference in cost and effect: the cost-effectiveness ratio and net monetary benefit (NMB). In Chapters 8 and 9, we explain concepts underlying quantification of sampling uncertainty around these point estimates (Chapter 8) and provide methods for the calculation of this uncertainty (Chapter 9).

In what follows, we define the cost-effectiveness ratio and NMB, we introduce the cost-effectiveness plane, a common method for depicting the difference in cost and effect; and we describe criteria for choosing between therapies when we focus on point estimates and ignore sampling uncertainty.

7.1. The cost-effectiveness ratio

One method for comparing the cost and effect of two therapies is to calculate an incremental cost-effectiveness ratio, which is defined as:

$$\frac{\text{Cost}_A - \text{Cost}_B}{\text{Effect}_A - \text{Effect}_B} = \frac{\Delta C}{\Delta Q} = \frac{C}{Q} \tag{7.1}$$

where Cost_A is the arithmetic mean cost for treatment group A; Cost_B is the arithmetic mean cost for treatment group B; Effect_A is the arithmetic mean effect for treatment group A; Effect_B is the arithmetic mean effect for treatment group B; ΔC and C equal the difference in cost; and ΔQ and Q equal the difference in effect.

7.1.1. **The cost-effectiveness plane**

The difference in cost and difference in effect is often depicted on the cost-effectiveness plane [1,2] (see Fig. 7.1). Incremental cost is plotted on the Y axis and incremental effect is plotted on the X axis. While some authors reverse the two, when the plane is constructed with the difference in cost on the Y axis, the slope of a ray from the origin to any cost–effect combination represents the cost-effectiveness ratio. Difference in cost and effect between two therapies can fall into one of four quadrants. A therapy can cost more and do more than another, in which case it lies in the upper right quadrant; it can cost less and do less (lower left quadrant); it can cost less and do more (lower right – or dominant – quadrant); or it can cost more and do less (upper left – or dominated – quadrant).

As drawn, the cost-effectiveness plane does not report each therapy's cost and effect, but instead reports the difference in cost and effect. Thus, we have subtracted the cost and effect of one therapy from the cost and effect of the other (in cases where we are comparing more than one therapy, we subtract one therapy's cost and effect from all other therapies' cost and effect). We can think of the origin of the cost-effectiveness plane as representing the

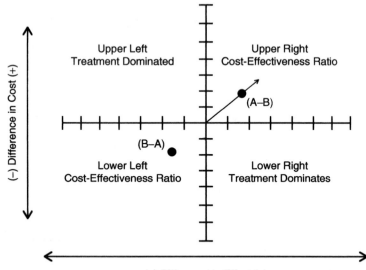

Fig. 7.1 The cost-effectiveness plane. Potential outcomes of the comparison of the difference in cost and effect. The X axis represents the difference in effect between the therapies; the Y axis represents the difference in cost between the therapies. Reproduced from Henry A Glick, Andrew H Briggs[t] and Daniel Polsky featured in Expert Rev. Pharmacoeconomics Outcomes Res. 1(1), (2001) with permission of Future Sciences Group.

therapy whose cost and effect has been subtracted from the other therapies (in this case, we have subtracted its cost and effect from itself, leaving both equal to 0).

If the therapy represented by the origin has the smaller point estimate for effect, the point estimate for the difference in cost and effect will fall in the upper or lower right quadrants of the graph. If the therapy represented by the origin has the larger point estimate for effect, the point estimate for the difference in cost and effect will fall in either the upper or lower left quadrants of the graph. If – as is usually assumed – our willingness to pay to gain health is symmetric with our willingness to save to give up health (see Chapter 9, p. **203**), our adoption decisions will be independent of the therapy we choose to represent the origin. If our willingness to pay and to save are not symmetric, we should use the origin to represent "current practice."

While choice of the therapy that is subtracted from the alternative affects the quadrant in which the point estimate for the difference in cost and effect falls, it does not affect which therapy is being described by the cost-effectiveness ratio. So long as we use the ratio to define the cost per unit of effect gained (e.g., cost per QALY gained), the point estimate for the cost-effectiveness ratio reports the trade-off between cost and effect for the therapy with the larger effect estimate in the denominator of the ratio. For example, Table 7.1 shows the ratio of the cost per QALY gained for therapy A, which costs 535 and yields 1.04 QALYs, compared to therapy B, which costs 500 and yields 1 QALY. If we subtract therapy B from therapy A, the resulting cost-effectiveness ratio, 875, indicates that when we move from the origin to the point in the upper right quadrant in Fig. 7.1, we incur a cost of 875 for each additional QALY yielded by therapy A. If in Table 7.1 we subtract A from B, on the other hand, the resulting cost-effectiveness ratio, 875, indicates that when we move from the point in the lower left quadrant to the origin in Fig. 7.1, we continue to incur a cost of 875 for each additional QALY yielded by A.

Conversely, if we define the ratio as the savings per unit of effect sacrificed, the point estimate for the cost-effectiveness ratio reports the trade-off between cost and effect for the therapy with the smaller effect estimate in the denominator of the ratio.

Table 7.1 The point estimate for the ratio of the cost per unit of effect gained reports the trade-off between cost and effect for the therapy with the larger point estimate for effect in the denominator of the ratio

Calculated difference	Cost-effectiveness ratio
A – B	$(535 - 500)/(1.04 - 1) = 35/0.04 = 875/QALY$
B – A	$(500 - 535)/(1 - 1.04) = -35/-0.04 = 875/QALY$

When we are evaluating the point estimate for the cost-effectiveness ratio, we thus require only three pieces of information to understand the value message: the cost-effectiveness ratio, the therapy with the larger point estimate for effect, and our willingness to pay. If the ratio of the cost per unit of effect gained is lower than our willingness to pay, it provides evidence supporting the value of the therapy with the larger point estimate for effect; if the ratio is greater than our willingness to pay, it provides evidence against the value of this therapy.

Foreshadowing our discussion in Chapter 8, the fact that the cost-effectiveness ratio reports the trade-off between cost and effect for the therapy with the larger effect estimate in the denominator of the ratio can lead to counterintuitive confidence limits for the cost-effectiveness ratio. If, for example, the 0.04 difference in effect described in Table 7.1 is not significant, one confidence limit for the ratio refers to the case where A is likely to be more effective than B, whereas the other limit refers to the case where B is likely to be more effective than A. Thus, as we have defined the cost-effectiveness ratio, each of the two limits will actually be referring to a different therapy, and they both will not be describing the additional cost we incur for an additional unit of effect yielded by therapy A.

7.1.2. **Choosing among therapies**

Most commonly, we make adoption decisions by comparing a therapy's cost-effectiveness ratio to a predefined standard (i.e., a maximum acceptable cost-effectiveness ratio or maximum willingness to pay), for example 30,000 or 50,000 per QALY. We adopt this convention for selecting therapies in our discussion below. In some jurisdictions, there may be general agreement on the value of this maximum willingness to pay [3–5]; in others, there is not [6]. At the level of the individual patient, rather than at the policy level, there is a growing body of research that uses measures of QALY diminutions for a condition and willingness to pay for a cure for that condition to quantify the value of a QALY [7–12]. Currently, the results from these studies are very variable.

If we wish to select therapies but have not quantified sampling uncertainty, the following five guidelines summarize current recommendations:

(1) If a therapy has a significantly larger cost and effect than the alternative, adopt the therapy if the point estimate for the cost-effectiveness ratio and cost-effectiveness ratios from sensitivity analysis are generally below our maximum willingness to pay; reject the therapy if these ratios are generally above our maximum willingness to pay.

(2) If a therapy has a significantly smaller cost and has a significantly larger effect than the alternative (both as point estimates and in sensitivity analysis), adopt this dominant therapy. If the therapy has a significantly larger cost and a significantly smaller effect, reject this dominated therapy.

In neither case is there a need to formally compare cost and effect by use of a cost-effectiveness ratio.

(3) If the therapies are not significantly different in effect, adopt the therapy with the significantly lower cost (cost-minimization). As with criterion 2, there is no need to formally compare cost and effect by use of cost-effectiveness ratio.

(4) If the therapies are not significantly different in cost, adopt the therapy with the significantly larger effect (effect-maximization), again without the assistance of the calculation of a cost-effectiveness ratio.

(5) If the therapies fail to differ significantly in both their cost and effect, there is no reason to evaluate cost-effectiveness because there is no evidence that the therapies differ.

In other words, when we do not account for sampling uncertainty, there is one case in which we need to calculate cost-effectiveness ratios for adoption decisions (significantly larger cost and effect), and four cases where we need not (significantly smaller cost and significantly larger effect, or lack of significant difference for one or both of the cost and effect measures). Once we account for sampling uncertainty surrounding these estimates, we will see in Chapter 9 that the last three of these recommendations are turned on their head.

The discussion above focuses on comparing two therapies. However, a ratio exists for every pair of therapies that is evaluated in a trial. When more than two therapies are compared, our goal is to identify the therapy that has both the largest measure of effectiveness and an acceptable cost-effectiveness ratio. Table 7.2 provides a summary of a method for identifying this therapy. See Box 7.1 for a worked out example.

Finally, other potential methods for choosing among therapies include comparison of the cost-effectiveness ratio with other accepted and rejected interventions (e.g., against league tables [14,15]). Alternatively, in theory, if we are able to derive indifference curves that trade-off health and cost, we would be able to determine whether the adoption of a therapy moves us to a lower or higher curve.

7.2. Net benefit

Net benefit [16] is a composite measure (part cost-effectiveness, part cost-benefit analysis) that is derived by rearranging the cost-effectiveness decision rule:

$$W > \frac{\text{Cost}_A - \text{Cost}_B}{\text{Effect}_A - \text{Effect}_B} = \frac{C}{Q}, \tag{7.2}$$

where W is the willingness to pay (e.g., 30,000 or 50,000). Net benefit transforms the comparison of cost and effect from ratio to linear values.

Table 7.2 Identification of the therapy with an acceptable ratio when more than two therapies are compared

(1)	Rank order therapies in ascending order of either effect or cost (the final ordering of the nondominated therapies will be the same whichever rank ordering you choose).
(2)	Eliminate therapies that have increased cost and reduced effect compared with at least one other therapy (referred to as strong dominance).
(3)	Compute incremental cost-effectiveness ratios for each of the remaining adjacent pair of therapies (e.g., between the therapies rank ordered 1 and 2; between the therapies rank ordered 2 and 3; etc.)
(4)	Eliminate therapies that have a smaller effect but a larger cost-effectiveness ratio compared to the next highest ranked therapy (referred to as extended or weak dominance).
(5)	Recalculate the incremental cost-effectiveness ratios for each remaining adjacent pair of therapies (steps 4 and 5 may need to be repeated).
(6)	Select the option with the largest incremental cost-effectiveness ratio that is less than the maximum willingness to pay.

Box 7.1 Identifying the cost-effective therapy when more than two therapies are compared

Suppose 6 strategies for screening for colorectal cancer have the following discounted costs and discounted life expectancies.

Screening strategy*	Cost	Life expectancy
No screening (S1)	1052	17.348
Sig,Q10 (S2)	1288	17.378
Sig,Q5 (S3)	1536	17.387
U+Sig,Q10 (S4)	1810	17.402
C,Q10 (S5)	2028	17.396
U+Sig,Q5 (S6)	2034	17.407

Source: Frazier et al. [13].
*Sig = Sigmoidoscopy
U = Unrehydrated fecal occult blood test;
C = Colonoscopy; Q10 every 10 years; Q5 every 5 years.

Step 1: Rank order therapies in ascending order of life expectancy.

Screening strategy	Cost	Life expectancy
S1	1052	17.348
S2	1288	17.378

Box 7.1 Identifying the cost-effective therapy when more than two therapies are compared *(continued)*

S3	1536	17.387
S5	2028	17.396
S4	1810	17.402
S6	2034	17.407

Step 2: Eliminate S5 because it has a larger cost and smaller effect than S4.

Screening strategy	Cost	Life expectancy
S1	1052	17.348
S2	1288	17.378
S3	1536	17.387
~~S5~~	~~2028~~	~~17.396~~
S4	1810	17.402
S6	2034	17.407

Step 3: Compute incremental cost-effectiveness ratios for each of the remaining adjacent pair of therapies.

Comparison	Cost per year of life saved
S2 versus S1	7850
S3 versus S2	27,550
S4 versus S3	18,250
S6 versus S4	44,800

Step 4: Eliminate S3 because the ratio for S4 versus S3 is smaller than the ratio for S3 versus S2, and S4 is more effective than S3.

Comparison	Cost per year of life saved
S2 versus S1	7850
~~S3 versus S2~~	~~27,550~~
S4 versus S3	18,250
S6 versus S4	44,800

Box 7.1 Identifying the cost-effective therapy when more than two therapies are compared (continued)

Step 5: Recalculate the incremental cost-effectiveness ratios for each of the remaining adjacent pair of therapies.

Comparison	Cost per year of life saved
S2 versus S1	7850
S4 versus S2	21,750
S6 versus S4	44,800

A more complete version of this table, with cost, incremental cost, effect, incremental effect, and incremental cost-effectiveness ratios is given below.

Screening strategy	Cost	ΔC	Life expectancy	ΔLE	$\Delta C/\Delta LE$
No screening (S1)	1052	–	17.348	–	–
Sig,Q10 (S2)	1288	236	17.378	0.030	7850
U+Sig,Q10 (S4)	1810	522	17.402	0.024	21,750
U+Sig,Q5 (S6)	2034	224	17.407	0.005	44,800

Step 6: Select the strategy with the largest incremental cost-effectiveness ratio that is less than the maximum willingness to pay. For example, if one's maximum willingness to pay is less than 7850, choose S1; if it is between 7850 and 21,750, choose S2; if it is between 21,750 and 44,800, choose S4; and if it is greater than 44,800, choose S6.

Two forms of the net benefit expression can be constructed depending on the rearrangement of this expression. For example, it can be constructed on the cost scale, in which case it is known as net monetary benefit (NMB)

$$(WQ) - C$$

Alternatively, net health benefit (NHB) can be constructed on the health outcome scale:

$$Q - (C/W)$$

In the following discussion, we principally refer to NMB rather than NHB, in part because NHB has the potential disadvantage of being undefined when W equals 0.

Whichever form of the net benefit expression is chosen, we should adopt therapies with net benefit greater than 0 (i.e., therapies with incremental cost-effectiveness ratios that are less than W). Given that not all decision-making bodies have an agreed upon maximum willingness to pay, we routinely estimate net benefit over the range of policy-relevant values of the willingness to pay.

Net benefit is defined on the cost-effectiveness plane by a family of lines, each with a slope equal to W (see Fig. 7.2). Each line represents a single value of net benefit, which for NMB is defined by multiplying −1 times the value of the line's intercept. NMB equals minus the intercept because the NMB equation represents the formula for a line in which W equals the slope and $-C$ is the intercept and because at the intercept, the difference in QALYs is 0, so W times Q equals 0 and we are left with $-C$. When these same lines are interpreted as NHB, their Q value is defined by the value of the point where the lines intersect the horizontal axis.

NMB lines that pass through the origin have a value of 0. Lines below and to the right of the line where net benefit equals 0 line have positive net benefits, while those above and to the left have negative net benefits.

NMB, like the cost-effectiveness ratio, is constructed by use of the difference in arithmetic mean cost and effect (by multiplying W times Q and subtracting C). The equations in Table 7.3 show that we can expand the NMB equation,

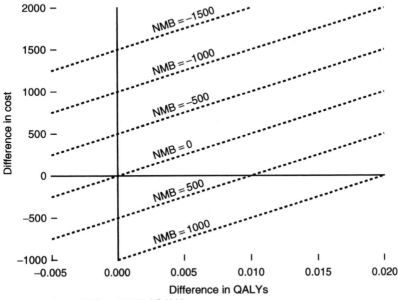

Willingness to pay (W) = 50,000 / QALY

Fig. 7.2 Net monetary benefit (NMB) lines plotted for a willingness to pay of 50,000 per QALY.

Table 7.3 Equivalence of NMB calculated by use of differences in arithmetic means versus calculated individually for each participant in the trial

(1)	$(WQ) - C > 0$
(2)	$\{W\ [(\Sigma_i\ E_{Ai}/N_A] - (\Sigma_i\ E_{Bi}/N_B)]\} - \{(\Sigma_i\ C_{Ai}/N_A) - (\Sigma_i\ C_{Bi}/N_B)\} > 0$
(3)	$(\Sigma_i\ W\ E_{Ai}/N_A) - (\Sigma_i\ W\ E_{Bi}/N_B) > (\Sigma_i\ C_{Ai}/N_A) - (\Sigma_i\ C_{Bi}/N_B)$
(4)	$(\Sigma_i\ W\ E_{Ai}/N_A) - (\Sigma_i\ C_{Ai}/N_A) > (\Sigma_i\ W\ E_{Bi}/N_B) - (\Sigma_i\ C_{Bi}/N_B)$
(5)	$\Sigma_i([W\ E_{Ai}] - C_{Ai})/N_A > \Sigma_i([W\ E_{Bi}] - C_{Bi})/N_B$
(6)	$\{\Sigma_i[(W\ E_{Ai}) - C_{Ai}]/N_A\} - \{\Sigma_i[(W\ E_{Bi}) - C_{Bi}]/N_B\} > 0$

where E_{Ai} is the effect for participant i among those who receive therapy A; N_A is the number of participants who receive therapy A; E_{Bi} is the effect for participant i among those who receive therapy B; N_B is the number of participants who receive therapy B; C_{Ai} is the cost for participant i among those who receive therapy A; and C_{Bi} is the cost for participant i among those who receive therapy B.

when written by use of arithmetic means, such that we can also construct NMB by multiplying W times each participant's effect and subtracting each participant's cost. In doing so, each participant (i) has a monetary benefit (NMB$_i$ = [WQ_i] – C_i) in the same way that each participant has an estimate of cost or effect. Thus, one potential advantage of NMB compared with cost-effectiveness ratios is that we can directly compare the difference in arithmetic mean monetary benefits between treatment groups to determine NMB by use of the same types of univariate and multivariable methods that we have already described in Chapter 5 [17].

7.2.1. Choosing among therapies

If we are using NMB to choose between therapies, the analog of the cost-effectiveness selection guidelines is to select the therapy with the largest NMB when we calculate NMB by use of the maximum willingness to pay. As with the five guidelines for choice by use of cost-effectiveness ratios, if we wish to select therapies but have not quantified sampling uncertainty, we must calculate NMB when a therapy has a significantly larger cost and effect than the alternative. In this case, we should adopt the therapy with the greater NMB. For the other four potential outcomes, significantly lower cost and significantly larger effect (dominance), no significant difference in effect but significantly lower cost (cost minimization), no significant difference in cost, but significantly larger effect (effect maximization), and no significant difference in cost and effect, selection can be made without the calculation of NMB.

7.3. **Summary**

We can compare our estimates of the difference in cost and effect by use of either a cost-effectiveness ratio or NMB. These two methods represent transformations of one another: we evaluate value either by comparing the resulting cost-effectiveness ratio to our willingness to pay or by building our willingness to pay into the construction of NMB and comparing the resulting NMB to 0.

Much of the information about value for the cost is communicated by plotting the distribution of the difference in cost and effect on the cost-effectiveness plane. We recommend plotting the difference in effect on the Y axis and the difference in cost on the X axis. Ratios of cost per unit of effect gained that are depicted on this graph represent the additional cost per unit of additional effect for the therapy with the larger estimate of effectiveness in the denominator of the ratio.

Finally, so long as we evaluate point estimates for the cost-effectiveness ratio or NMB alone, there is only one case where we need to calculate these quantities: when the difference in cost and effect are significantly greater than 0. When it is not the case that both are greater than 0, guidelines for point estimate determinations of value suggest we choose the significantly more effective or less costly therapy and need not further compare cost and effect.

References

1. **Anderson JP, Bush JW, Chen M, Dolenc D.** Policy space areas and properties of benefit cost/utility analysis. *JAMA*. 1986; 255: 794–5.
2. **Black WC.** The CE plane: a graphic representation of cost-effectiveness. *Med Decis Making* 1990; 10: 212–4.
3. **Towse A.** What is NICE's threshold? An external view, Chapter 2. In *Cost-effectiveness Thresholds: Economic and Ethical Issues*, edited by N. Devlin and A. Towse. Kings Fund/Office for Health Economics: London, 2002.
4. **Devlin N, Parkin D.** Does NICE have a cost-effectiveness threshold and what other factors influence its decisions? A binary choice analysis. *Health Econ.* 2004; 13: 437–52.
5. **George B, Harris A, Mitchell A.** Cost-effectiveness analysis and the consistency of decision making. Evidence from pharmaceutical reimbursement in Australia (1991 to 1996). *Pharmacoeconomics* 2001; 19: 1103–9.
6. **Hirth RA, Chernew ME, Miller E, Fendrick M, Weissert WG.** Willingness to pay for a quality-adjusted life year: in search of a standard. *Med Dec Making* 2000; 20: 332–42.
7. **Blumenschein B, Johannesson M.** Relationship between quality of life instruments, health state utilities, and willingness to pay in patients with asthma. *Ann Allergy Asthma Immunol.* 1998; 80: 189–94.
8. **Byrne MM, O'Malley K, Suarez-Almazor ME.** Willingness to pay per quality-adjusted life year in a study of knee osteoarthritis. *Med Decis Making* 2005; 25: 655–66.

9. King JT, Styn MA, Tsevat J, Roberts MS. "Perfect health" versus "disease free": the impact of anchor point choice on the measurement of preferences and the calculation of disease-specific disutilities. *Med Decis Making* 2003; 23: 212–25.

10. King JT, Tsevat J, Lave JR, Roberts MS. Willingness to pay for a quality-adjusted life year: implications for societal health care resource allocation. *Med Decis Making* 2005; 25: 667–77.

11. Lundberg L, Johannesson M, Siverdahl M, Hermansson C, Lindberg M. Quality of life, health-state utilities and willingness to pay in patients with psoriasis and atopic eczema. *Br J Dermatol.* 1999; 141: 1067–75.

12. Voruganti LNP, Awad AG, Oyewumi LK, Cortese L, Zirul S, Dhawan R. Assessing health utilities in schizophrenia. *Pharmacoeconomics* 2000; 17: 273–86.

13. Frazier AL, Colditz GA, Fuchs CS, Kuntz KM. Cost-effectiveness of screening for colorectal cancer in the general population. *JAMA.* 2000; 284: 1954–61.

14. Drummond M, Torrance G, Mason J. Cost-effectiveness league tables: more harm than good? *Soc Sci Med.* 1993; 37: 33–40.

15. Mauskopf J, Rutten F, Schonfeld W. Cost-effectiveness league tables. *Pharmacoeconomics* 2003; 21: 991–1000.

16. Stinnett AA, Mullahy J. Net health benefits: a new framework for the analysis of uncertainty in cost-effectiveness analysis. *Med Decis Making* 1998; 18: S65–80.

17. Hoch JS, Briggs AH, Willan AR. Something old, something new, something borrowed, something blue: a framework for the marriage of health econometrics and cost-effectiveness analysis. *Health Econ.* 2002; 11: 415–30.

Chapter 8

Understanding sampling uncertainty: the concepts

A common goal of an economic analysis in medicine is to identify when we can be confident that one medical therapy is "good value" compared to another. One of the threats to such confidence is that the economic result observed in an experiment may not truly reflect the result in the population. This is because it is the result of a single sample drawn from a population: had one repeated the experiment with a different sample from the population, one would have obtained a different point estimate. This form of uncertainty is referred to as sampling (or stochastic) uncertainty. One approach that is commonly used to address this threat is to use the data from the experiment to identify when we can be confident about the value for the cost of one or the other therapies and when we cannot be confident that they differ.

In this chapter, we demonstrate the quantification and interpretation of sampling uncertainty by use of confidence intervals for cost-effectiveness ratios, confidence intervals for net monetary benefit (NMB), and acceptability curves. We also identify and interpret hard cases for these three methods. In doing so, we identify three distinct patterns of results into which all experiments fall. In Chapter 9, we introduce methods of calculation, identify when the three distinct patterns of experiments are observed; provide methods for calculation of sample size and power for evaluation of economic outcomes; and describe revisions to decision rules for choosing therapies that are prompted by consideration of sampling uncertainty.

8.1. Sampling uncertainty for clinical outcomes

In many ways, methods used to evaluate sampling uncertainty for economic evaluation are similar to methods used to evaluate sampling uncertainty for clinical outcomes of experiments. In both cases, we determine the point estimate in the sample; we quantify sampling uncertainty; and we compare it against a decision threshold.

For example, if illness occurs in 15 out of 150 participants who receive one form of prevention while it occurs in 30 out of 150 who receive an alternative form, we would conclude that the odds ratio for disease is 0.44 ((15×120)/(30×135)) for the first form of prevention compared to the alternative and that its 95% confidence interval is 0.23–0.86. All three values are less than 1, which represents the decision threshold for determining whether an intervention is effective when measured by use of odds ratios; thus, we can be 95% confident that the first form of prophylaxis is more effective than the alternative form.

One can also evaluate the difference in risk for disease between the two forms of prevention. The risk for disease is 10% for the first form of prevention, and it is 20% for the second form. The risk difference is 10%; the 95% confidence interval for the risk difference is 0.016–0.184. Because all three values are greater than 0, which represents the decision threshold for determining whether an intervention is effective when measured by risk difference, we can be 95% confident that the first form of prophylaxis is more effective than the alternative form.

If, on the other hand, the 95% confidence interval for the odds ratio had included 1 (a p value > 0.05) or the 95% confidence interval for the risk difference had included 0, we could not be 95% confident that the two forms of prophylaxis differ in their effectiveness.

8.2. **Sampling uncertainty for economic outcomes**

We follow similar steps when evaluating sampling uncertainty for the comparison of cost and effect. For example, we can express sampling uncertainty by use of confidence intervals for cost-effectiveness ratios [1,2]. In this case, we estimate the point estimate for the ratio; we estimate its 95% confidence interval; and we determine whether we can be 95% confident that therapy A is good value by comparing the confidence interval to the decision threshold, which for cost-effectiveness analysis is our maximum willingness to pay for a unit of health outcome. If our maximum willingness to pay falls within the confidence interval, we cannot be confident that the two therapies differ in their cost effectiveness. If it falls outside the interval, we can be 95% confident that one of the therapies is cost effective compared to the other.

Alternatively, we might express sampling uncertainty by use of confidence intervals for NMB [3]. We again estimate the point estimate of NMB; we estimate its 95% confidence interval; and we determine whether we can be 95% confident that therapy A is good value by comparing the confidence interval to the decision threshold, which for NMB is 0.

Finally, we might express sampling uncertainty by use of an acceptability curve (described below).

8.3. **Differences in interpreting sampling uncertainty for clinical and economic outcomes**

While it is true that many of the same methods are used to evaluate sampling uncertainty for clinical and economic outcomes, there are at least two differences that exist as well. First, for differences in height or weight or differences in risk, there is little debate that the decision threshold is 0, i.e., confidence intervals for these differences that include 0 represent cases where we cannot be confident that the therapies differ and confidence intervals that exclude 0 represent cases where we can be confident. Similarly, for odds ratios and relative risks, there is little debate that the decision threshold is 1.0, i.e., confidence intervals for odds ratios and relative risks that include 1 represent cases where we cannot be confident and confidence intervals that exclude 1 represent cases where we can be confident.

As we have indicated earlier, jurisdictions exist in which there is much less agreement about the appropriate willingness to pay for a unit of health outcome. In fact, it is expected that the maximum willingness to pay can differ among decision makers, particularly in different decision-making jurisdictions, ranging from the micro level of different formularies to the macro level of decision-making bodies in different countries. Furthermore, it would not be inconsistent for a single decision maker to vary her maximum willingness to pay based on other features of the decision problem, such as if the health problem in question is immediately life threatening and incurable versus one that principally affects quality of life; if the therapy has a small budgetary impact, such as an orphan drug; if the condition strikes identifiable individuals rather than "statistical" individuals; or if the condition is self-imposed versus imposed by society.

Second, while it frequently may be stated that 95% confidence is arbitrary for judging clinical outcomes, there is near universal agreement among regulatory bodies and medical journals that this level of confidence is required for making a claim that two therapies differ clinically. Such agreement is less clear in the economics community, in which there is discussion about whether we need to have the same degree of confidence about health returns on our investments as we do about clinical outcomes. This idea that our confidence statements are only about money and thus are not the same as our confidence statements about health becomes blurred, however, when we are asked to give up health to save money in one area of medicine, because we believe the return on our investment will be greater in another area. Nevertheless, the conclusions we draw below apply whether we are seeking 95% confidence, 75% confidence, or even 1% confidence when making adoption decisions.

8.4. Experiment 1, a significant difference in effect yields a familiar pattern of results for the comparison of cost and effect

In what follows, we demonstrate the evaluation of sampling uncertainty for three different experiments. These experiments were selected because they span the three patterns of results we can observe for the comparison of cost and effect. Experiment 1 has a familiar pattern of results, and its interpretation is most straightforward. Experiments 2 and 3 have less familiar patterns of results. While the confidence statements that we can make about these latter experiments are as interpretable as the confidence statements we can make about experiment 1, these less familiar patterns of results may stretch the reader's understanding of what it means to be a confidence interval.

To state our conclusions for these three experiments in advance, first, if our goal is to determine whether we can be confident, given our maximum willingness to pay, that therapy A is good value compared to therapy B, that therapy A is not good value, or that we cannot be confident that the economic value of therapies A and B differs, confidence intervals for cost-effectiveness ratios, confidence intervals for NMB, and acceptability curves all yield the same conclusions. Second, the confidence limits for cost-effectiveness ratios provide decision makers with a concise set of information that allows them to determine if they can be confident about a therapy's value for the cost. Third, acceptability curves provide the added advantage of allowing decision makers to assess alternate levels of confidence if such alternative levels are of interest.

8.4.1. Experiment 1

Suppose you conducted an economic evaluation of two therapies and found that therapy A on average cost 1000 more than therapy B (SE, 325, $p = 0.002$); therapy A on average yielded 0.01 QALYs more than therapy B (SE, 0.001925, $p = 0.0000$); the correlation between the difference in cost and effect was -0.71; and there were 250 participants per group in the trial.

8.4.2. Confidence intervals for cost-effectiveness ratios

As with clinical outcomes, to evaluate value for the cost, we estimate a point estimate for the cost-effectiveness ratio of 100,000 (1000/0.01) per QALY. We next calculate a confidence interval for a cost-effectiveness ratio, which is most easily interpreted on the cost-effectiveness plane. Figure 8.1 shows the confidence interval for the cost-effectiveness ratio for experiment 1. The cloud of + signs represents the joint distribution of the difference in cost and QALYs for the experiment. Confidence limits are defined by lines through the origin

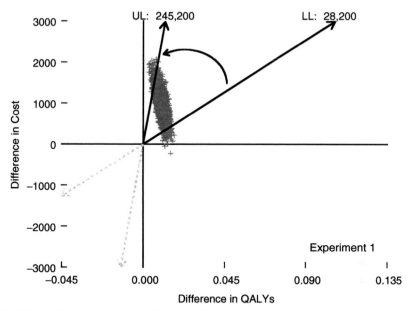

Fig. 8.1 Confidence interval for the cost-effectiveness ratio observed in experiment 1.

that each exclude $\alpha/2$ of the distribution of the difference in cost and effect, i.e., for 95% confidence – which will be the level of confidence used for the remainder of this book – that each exclude 2.5% of the distribution. In the figure, 2.5% of the distribution of the difference in cost and effect falls below and to the right of the dashed and solid line with a slope of 28,200 (rounded to the nearest 100) representing the lower limit; 2.5% of the distribution falls above and to the left of the dashed and solid line with a slope of 245,200 (rounded to the nearest 100) that represents the upper limit. The part of the joint distribution that is included within the limits is the region in the upper right quadrant that falls between 28,200 and 245,200.

For experiments with this pattern of results, if our maximum willingness to pay is less than the lower limit, we can be 95% confident that therapy A is not good value, i.e., not cost-effective, compared to therapy B. For example, if our maximum willingness to pay is 10,000, then there is less than a one-tailed 2.5% chance that A's cost-effectiveness ratio is less than this willingness to pay, i.e., two-tailed 95% confidence that it is greater than 10,000. If our maximum willingness to pay falls between the limits, we cannot be 95% confident that the economic value of therapy A differs from therapy B. Finally, if our maximum willingness to pay is greater than the upper limit, we can be 95% confident that therapy A is good value compared to therapy B. For example, if our maximum willingness to pay is 250,000, then there is less than a one-tailed

2.5% chance that A's cost-effectiveness ratio is greater than this willingness to pay, i.e., two-tailed 95% confidence that it is less than 250,000.

8.4.3. Confidence intervals for net monetary benefit (NMB)

Alternatively, we might compare cost and effect by use of NMB. Recall that we can be confident that an intervention is cost effective if we can be confident that NMB calculated by use of the maximum willingness to pay is greater than 0.

As with clinical outcomes and cost-effectiveness ratios, we calculate a point estimate for NMB, but unlike these other two outcomes, given that NMB depends upon our willingness to pay (W), we calculate point estimates for each value of W that may be relevant. We express sampling uncertainty around NMB by use of confidence intervals, again with the understanding that each point estimate has its own confidence interval. Finally, we determine whether we can be confident that the two therapies differ if the confidence interval calculated for the maximum willingness to pay excludes 0, which is the decision threshold for determining if an intervention is net monetarily beneficial.

For a willingness to pay of 50,000, the point estimate of NMB for experiment 1 is −500 ((50,000 × 0.01) − 1000). Figure 8.2 depicts the construction of 95% confidence intervals for a willingness to pay of 50,000 for this experiment. The cloud of points in the figure is identical to the cloud shown in Fig. 8.1; the only difference is that in Fig. 8.2, we have zoomed in on the region of cost between −500 and 2500 and the region of QALYs between −0.005 and 0.02. As we indicated in Chapter 7, when drawn on the cost-effectiveness plane, the NMB for each point is defined by multiplying −1 times the intercept of the line with a slope 50,000 that intersects the point. In the figure, we show a histogram of NMB. We identify the 95% confidence limits by identifying the intercepts of lines that exclude 2.5% of the tails of this distribution. The lower limit is −1×1284 (−1284); the upper limit is −1×−284 (284). Thus, if our maximum willingness to pay is 50,000, the confidence interval includes 0 and the result of experiment 1 does not allow us to be 95% confident that the two therapies differ from one another.

If, on the other hand, our maximum willingness to pay is not 50,000, this confidence interval need not provide information for the determination of whether we can be confident about the value for the cost of the two therapies. For example, for a willingness to pay of 10,000, the confidence interval for NMB ranges from −1566 to −234, in which case we can be 95% confident that A is not good value compared to B. If our willingness to pay is 250,000, the confidence interval for NMB ranges between 31 and 2969, in which case we can be 95% confident that A is good value compared to B.

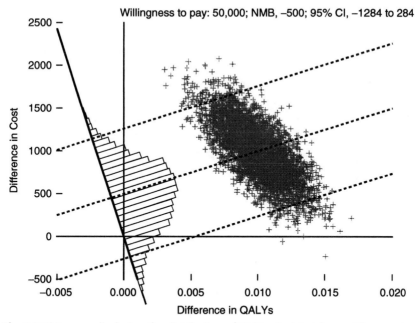

Fig. 8.2 Histogram displaying the distribution of NMB calculated for a willingness to pay of 50,000. We can construct 95% confidence intervals by identifying the intercepts of lines with slope equal to 50,000 that exclude 2.5% of the lower and upper tails of the distribution.

We normally display point estimates and confidence intervals for NMBs calculated for a range of willingnesses to pay by use of a NMB graph like the one shown in Fig. 8.3. The solid line in the figure represents the point estimates for NMB for willingnesses to pay that range from 0 to 400,000. The lower dashed line represents the lower limit of NMB; the upper dashed line represents the upper limit.

Intersections of the confidence limits for NMB with the X axis, which in this example are represented by the superimposed lines at 28,200 and 245,200, define the boundaries between the range of willingnesses to pay where we can be confident that therapy A is not cost-effective compared to therapy B, the range where we cannot be confident that the value of the two therapies differ, and the range of willingnesses to pay where we can be confident that therapy A is cost-effective compared to therapy B. The boundary between the first two ranges is 28,200. Below this willingness to pay, the lower and upper confidence limits are negative, the interval does not include 0, and we can be 95% confident that therapy A is not good value. The boundary between the second two ranges is 245,200. Above this willingness to pay, the lower and upper limits are positive, the interval does not include 0, and we can be 95% confident that

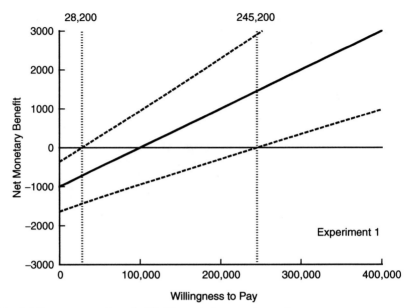

Fig. 8.3 Net monetary benefit (NMB) graph for experiment 1.

therapy A is good value. The range where we cannot be confident that the two therapies differ is between 28,200 and 245,200. In this range, one of the limits is positive; one is negative; and the interval includes the decision threshold, 0.

If you compare the boundaries between these three ranges to the confidence limits for the cost-effectiveness ratio reported in Fig. 8.1, you will find that they are one and the same. This identity is not an accident. As Heitjan [4] has shown, we can derive the formula for parametric confidence intervals for cost-effectiveness ratios (see Chapter 9, equation 9.1, p. **180**) by solving the NMB confidence limit equation (see Chapter 9, equation 9.3, p. **184**) for the willingnesses to pay that yield NMB limits that equal 0. Thus, in experiments with this familiar pattern of results, confidence intervals for cost-effectiveness ratios and confidence intervals for NMB yield identical information about when we can and cannot be confident that one medical therapy is cost-effective compared to another.

Finally, NMB curves like those in Fig. 8.3 contain substantially more information than simply reporting the NMB and 95% confidence intervals for varying willingnesses to pay [2]. As seen in Fig. 8.4, the NMB curve cuts the vertical axis at $-C$ (a), because at the vertical axis W equals 0, which when multiplied by Q leaves NMB equal to $0-C$. The NMB confidence limit curves cut the vertical axis at -1 times the confidence interval for C for the same reason. The NMB curve cuts the horizontal axis at the point estimate of the

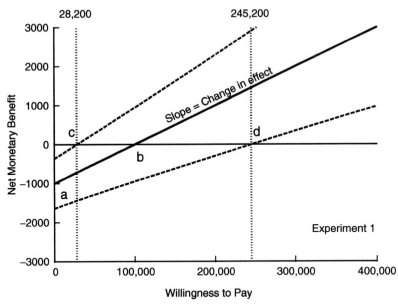

Fig. 8.4 Additional information contained in an NMB graph.

cost-effectiveness ratio (b) because when W equals C/Q, the NMB equation equals 0. The slope of the NMB curve equals Q because the NMB equation defines a line with slope Q and intercept $-C$. Finally, as already noted, the curves defining the upper and lower confidence limits of NMB intersect the horizontal axis at the lower and upper limits of the confidence interval for the cost-effectiveness ratio. For example, in Fig. 8.4, the NMB limit curves intersect the X axis at 28,200 (upper limit curve) (c) and 245,200 (lower limit curve) (d) which equal the confidence limits reported in Fig. 8.1.

8.4.4. Acceptability curves

A third method for evaluating sampling uncertainty for economic outcomes is by use of acceptability curves [5–8]. We construct acceptability curves by calculating the probability that the estimated cost-effectiveness ratio falls below specified values of willingness to pay. The acceptability criterion is defined on the cost-effectiveness plane as a line passing through the origin with a slope equal to the willingness to pay (see Fig. 8.5). The proportion of the distribution of the difference in cost and effect that falls below and to the right of this line – i.e., the lower right side of the upper right quadrant, the lower right quadrant, and the lower right side of the lower left quadrant – is "acceptable" (i.e., has positive NMB). The proportion that is above and to the left of this line is "unacceptable."

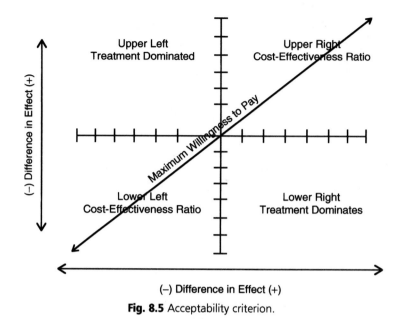

Fig. 8.5 Acceptability criterion.

As with NMB, given that there is no agreed upon maximum willingness to pay for use in the evaluation of medical therapies, we routinely estimate the probability of acceptability over the policy relevant range of values of willingness to pay, for example we might vary the slope of the line defining the willingness to pay in Fig. 8.5 from the horizontal through to the vertical. Plotting the proportion of the distribution of the difference in cost and effect that falls within the acceptable region of the cost-effectiveness plane as a function of the willingness to pay results in what is referred to as the cost-effectiveness acceptability curve. The X axis of this curve represents potential values for the willingness to pay, and the Y axis represents the proportion of the joint distribution that is acceptable. The acceptability curve for experiment 1 is shown in Fig. 8.6.

Evaluation of the height of the curve at willingnesses to pay of 28,200 and 245,200 provides insight into the statements of confidence that can be derived from acceptability curves. As with 95% confidence intervals, willingness to pay of 28,200 and 245,200 each exclude 2.5% of the distribution. When the height of the acceptability curve is below 2.5% (28,200), we can be 95% confident that therapy A is not good value compared with therapy B; when its height is above 97.5% (245,200), we can be 95% confident that it is good value compared to B; and when its height is between 2.5 and 97.5%, we cannot be 95% confident that the two therapies differ from one another. These are the same statements of confidence we derived by use of confidence intervals for cost-effectiveness ratios and confidence intervals for NMB.

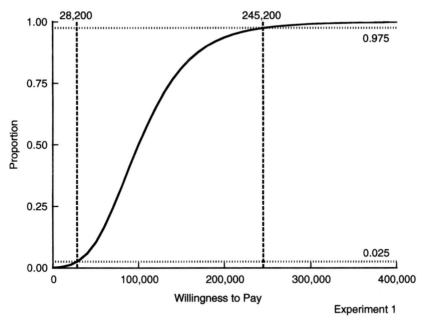

Fig. 8.6 Acceptability curve for experiment 1.

Again, the fact that the confidence statements we derive from the acceptability curve are the same as those we derive from the other two methods for quantifying sampling uncertainty is not an accident. We can derive the formula for parametric acceptability curves (see Chapter 9, equation 9.4, p. **185**) from the parametric formulas for either confidence limits for cost-effectiveness ratios or confidence limits for NMB. All three methods are simple transformations of one another. The acceptability curve has the added advantage that it allows us to make statements about varying levels of confidence. For example, when the curve has a height of 50%, we have 0% confidence that the two therapies differ. When it has a height less than or equal to 5% or greater than or equal to 95%, we can be 90% confident that therapy A is not good value (5%) or is good value (95%), etc.

Also, as with the NMB graph, the acceptability curve contains substantially more information than simply reporting the probability that a therapy's cost-effectiveness ratio falls below varying willingnesses to pay [2]. As seen in Fig. 8.7, the curve cuts the vertical axis, where the willingness to pay is 0, at the p value (one sided) for the difference in cost (a). This is because the fraction of the distribution of the difference in cost and effect that falls above and below the X axis on the cost-effectiveness plane defines a one-sided test of the difference in cost. For parametric acceptability curves, the 50% point corresponds

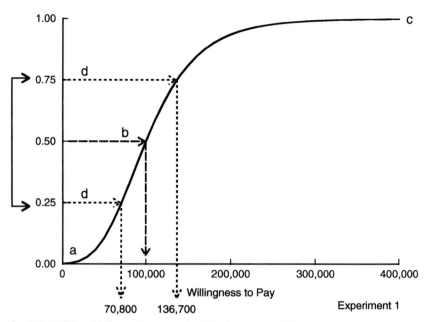

Fig. 8.7 Additional information contained in the acceptability curve.

to the point estimate of the cost-effectiveness ratio (b). As the willingness to pay approaches ∞, the curve asymptotically approaches 1 minus the p value (one-sided) for the effect difference (c), because the fraction of the distribution of the difference in cost and effect that falls to the left and right of the Y axis of the cost-effectiveness plane defines a one-sided test of the difference in effect. Finally, cutting α % from either end of the vertical axis and using the curve to map these values on to the horizontal willingness to pay axis defines the $(1-2\alpha)$% confidence interval for the cost-effectiveness ratio. For example, (d) defines the 50% confidence interval for the cost-effectiveness ratio, which ranges between 70,800 and 136,700.

8.4.5. Summary of findings from experiment 1

We refer to familiar findings like those in experiment 1 as pattern 1 findings. Pattern 1 findings occur when the difference in effect is significant ($p<\alpha$ for effect when we are seeking $1-\alpha$ confidence for determination of value for the cost). We know we are observing a pattern 1 finding when the confidence interval for the cost-effectiveness ratio excludes the Y axis, in which case the lower limit has the expected relationship of being less than the point estimate, which in turn has the expected relationship of being less than the upper limit. We also know we are observing this pattern of findings when both NMB

PATTERN #1

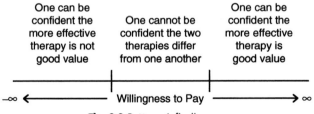

Fig. 8.8 Pattern 1 findings.

confidence limits intersect the decision threshold (0) once and when the acceptability curve intersects horizontal lines drawn at both 0.025 and 0.975 on the *Y* axis.

As shown in Fig. 8.8, if we consider willingnesses to pay that range from $-\infty$ to $+\infty$, pattern 1 findings are characterized by three ranges of willingness to pay for a unit of health outcome. On the left are those values of willingness to pay for which we can be confident that the therapy with the larger point estimate of effectiveness is not good value compared with the therapy with the smaller point estimate of effectiveness. In the middle are those values of willingness to pay for which we cannot be confident that the therapies differ. On the right are those values of willingness to pay for which we can be confident that the therapy with the larger point estimate of effectiveness is good value compared with the therapy with the smaller point estimate of effectiveness. In experiment 1, the boundaries between these ranges occur at 28,200 and 245,200.

Pattern 1 findings have the advantage that if we are confident that the more effective therapy is good value at a specific willingness to pay, we can be confident that it will be good value for all larger willingnesses to pay. If we are confident that it is not good value at a specific willingness to pay, we can be confident that it will not be good value for all smaller willingnesses to pay. Finally, if we cannot be confident that it is good value at a specific willingness to pay, we can be confident that there are both larger and (possibly negative) smaller willingnesses to pay where we can be confident in the therapy's value or the lack thereof.

Observation of pattern 1 findings is independent of the method we use to address sampling uncertainty. The three ranges of willingness to pay are defined identically by the confidence interval for the cost-effectiveness ratio, the confidence interval for NMB, and the acceptability curve. Observation of a pattern 1 finding, instead, depends upon the data as well as the level of confidence we desire. For example, all experiments that demonstrate pattern 1 findings for statements of 95% confidence will demonstrate other patterns for some – possibly extremely – higher levels of confidence.

Finally, as indicated in Fig. 8.8, pattern 1 findings are defined over the range of willingnesses to pay from $-\infty$ to $+\infty$. However, the policy relevant range of willingnesses to pay is bounded from below by 0. Thus, when plotting NMB confidence intervals or the acceptability curve, we will observe a left-truncated pattern whenever an intersection of a NMB confidence limit with the X axis or an intersection of the acceptability curve with horizontal lines drawn at 0.025 and 0.975 occurs where the willingness to pay is negative. For example, if the standard error for the difference in cost in experiment 1 had been 600 rather than 325, we would have observed only two ranges of willingness to pay on the NMB graph, one where we cannot be confident that the therapies differ and one where we can be confident that the therapy with the larger point estimate for effectiveness is good value compared with the alternative (see Fig. 8.9). We observe only two ranges because the NMB upper limit intersects the X axis at a willingness to pay of $-14,100$. Right truncation can also occur if we cap the plotted maximum willingness to pay at a finite value. In some cases, these truncations may be extreme enough that the resulting graphs will not provide sufficient information to determine whether we are observing a pattern 1 result or whether we are observing an experiment with a different pattern of results. Because confidence intervals for the cost-effectiveness ratio can be both positive and negative, such uncertainty never arises for them.

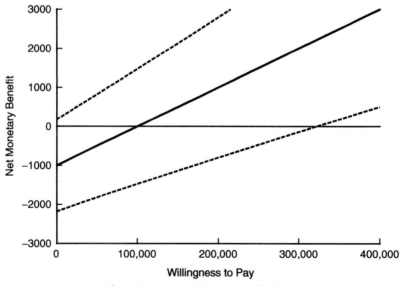

Fig. 8.9 A truncated pattern 1 finding.

8.5. **Experiment 2, No significant difference in effect yields an unfamiliar pattern of results for the comparison of cost and effect**

If all experiments had pattern 1 results, few if any of the debates about the benefits of confidence intervals for cost-effectiveness ratios, confidence intervals for NMB, and acceptability curves would arise. Given that not all experiments have significant differences in effect, however, not all experiments will have this pattern of results. In this section, we describe the first of two less familiar patterns of results.

One of the complications that arise when addressing sampling uncertainty for economic assessments is that when we draw two lines through the origin that each exclude 2.5% of the distribution of the difference in cost and effect, they can define the confidence limits for two or three very distinct sets of experiments. For example, Fig. 8.10A depicts the confidence interval for experiment 1, which we have already indicated, has confidence limits of 28,200 and 245,200. But Fig. 8.10B depicts the confidence interval for a second experiment, which we will call experiment 2, that also has confidence limits that, when rounded to the nearest 100, equal 28,200 and 245,200. Had we conducted this latter experiment, we might have found that therapy A on average cost 35 more than therapy B (SE, 0 777.5, p = 0.96); therapy A on average yielded 0.04 QALYs more than therapy B (SE, 0.0224, p = 0.37); the correlation between the difference in cost and effect was 0.706; and as with experiment 1, there were 250 participants per group in the trial. (In Chapter 9, we define a third experiment with equivalent limits which differs from the current two in that its point estimate for cost-effectiveness is greater than 245,200.)

While the limits for these two experiments are the same, they describe two very different, and in some sense diametrically opposed, therapy comparisons. First, except if one of the limits falls on the Y axis – which represents cost-effectiveness ratios equaling both $-\infty$ and $+\infty$) – one of the two confidence intervals must include the Y axis (in this case, experiment 2), whereas the other must fall into pattern 1 which does not include the Y axis (in this case, experiment 1). Thus, while the two experiments share the same limits, for experiment 1, the interval includes ratios that range between 28,200 and 245,200 and excludes ratios less than 28,200 (i.e., from $-\infty$ to 28,200) and greater than 245,200 (i.e., from 245,200 to ∞). For experiment 2, the interval excludes ratios that range between 28,200 and 245,200, and includes all other ratios ranging between $-\infty$ and $+\infty$.

Second, because confidence limits for cost-effectiveness ratios include the Y axis only when the difference in effect is not significant and exclude the

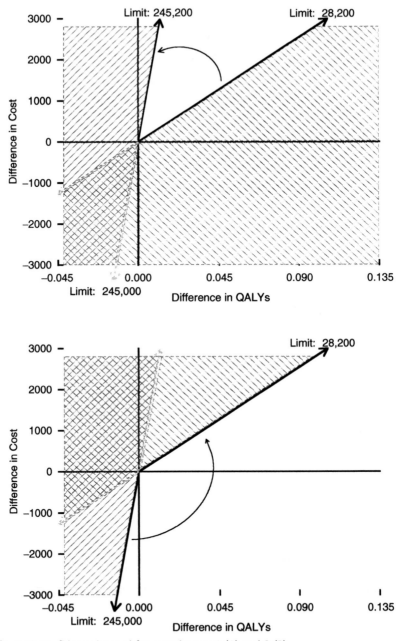

Fig. 8.10 Confidence interval for experiments 1 (A) and 2 (B).

Y axis only when the difference in effect is significant, in one of the experiments (in this case, experiment 2) we cannot be 95% confident that the two therapies differ in their effectiveness, whereas in the other experiment (in this case, experiment 1) one therapy's effectiveness must be significantly greater than the other's.

Third, except if one of the limits falls on the *X* axis, in one of the experiments cost must be significantly increased (in this case experiment 1), whereas in the other of the experiments, the cost difference cannot be significant (in this case experiment 2).

The union of the confidence intervals for these two experiments include all real numbers between $-\infty$ and $+\infty$ (i.e., $-\infty$ to 28,200 is included in experiment 2's interval; 28,200 to 245,200 is included in experiment 1's interval; and 245,200 to ∞ is included in experiment 2's interval). The intersection of the two confidence intervals is limited to the two confidence limits themselves (i.e., 28,200 and 245,200). Thus, fourth, except for the case where our maximum willingness to pay equals one of these two limits, the maximum willingness to pay must fall within the interval defined for one of the two experiments, in which case, we cannot be confident that the two therapies differ. Similarly, it must fall outside the interval defined for the other of the two experiments, in which case, we can be confident that one of the therapies is cost-effective compared to the other.

Given that the confidence limits are identical for these two very different sets of experiments, the challenge for confidence intervals for cost-effectiveness ratios is to provide a means for communicating which of the two experiments – one when effectiveness is significant and one when it is not – that we are observing when the reported confidence limits are 28,200 and 245,200. This challenge is not unique to confidence intervals for cost-effectiveness ratios alone. These two experiments also share intersections between the confidence limits for their respective NMBs and the *X* axis (i.e., at 28,200 and 245,200), and they share intersections between the acceptability curve and horizontal lines drawn at either 0.025 or 0.975 at 28,200 and 245,200. Thus, these latter two methods also share in the challenge of communicating which of the two experiments we are observing when reported intersections occur at 28,200 and 245,200.

The short answer to these challenges is that all three methods do something unexpected to communicate that we are no longer observing a pattern 1 result. Confidence intervals for cost-effectiveness ratios reverse the upper and lower limits, so that what was the upper limit for the pattern 1 experiment is now the lower limit for this second pattern of results and what was the lower limit is now the upper limit. Confidence limits for NMB still intersect the

X axis of the NMB graph at the lower and upper limits of the confidence interval for the cost-effectiveness ratio, but one of the NMB limits intersects this axis twice and the second NMB limit never intersects this axis. Finally, acceptability curves continue to intersect the decision thresholds twice, but they intersect one of the thresholds (either 0.025 or 0.975) twice and never intersect the second threshold. In the remainder of this section, we provide a detailed explanation of this short answer. If you are not interested in this detailed explanation, you may want to skip to Section 8.5.3 (see p. **169**).

8.5.1. **Confidence intervals for cost-effectiveness ratios**

The point estimate for the cost-effectiveness ratio in experiment 2 is 875 (35/0.04). Fig. 8.11 shows the confidence interval for the cost-effectiveness ratio. Here, 2.5% of the distribution falls above and to the left of the 245,200 limit; 2.5% falls above and to the left of the 28,200 limit.

Readers who are not familiar with confidence intervals for cost-effectiveness ratios that include the *Y* axis often find them counterintuitive. In what follows, we identify three of these counter-intuitive relationships and explain them. First, when we look at Fig. 8.11, the interval looks continuous without any gaps. Why do we say that the interval ranges from 28,200 to −∞ and from 245,200 to +∞ and has a gap between 28,200 and 245,200? Second, how is it

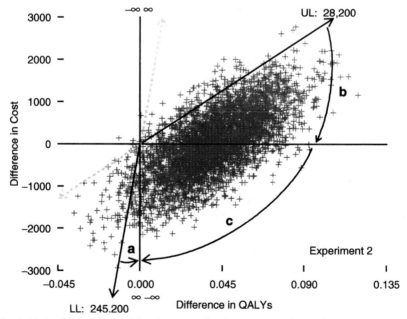

Fig. 8.11 Confidence interval for the cost-effectiveness ratio observed in experiment 2.

possible for the lower limit to be a larger number than the upper limit? Third, given the point estimate is in the center of the distribution of the difference in cost and effect, which in Fig. 8.11 is included within the confidence interval, how is it possible that the point estimate is not bounded by its limits?

1. Why does the confidence interval for the cost-effectiveness ratio look continuous on the cost-effectiveness plane, but have a gap between 28,200 and 245,200?

   To understand how the cost-effectiveness ratio can look continuous on the cost-effectiveness plane, yet have a gap, we must recognize that while the confidence region is continuous on the two-dimensional cost-effectiveness plane, when we collapse the result to the real number line it has several discontinuities, which all occur on the Y axis.

   For example, if we approach the Y axis from the left in the lower left quadrant, we are approaching a cost-effectiveness ratio of $+\infty$. That is because the numerator of the ratio, the difference in cost, is negative; the denominator of the ratio, the difference in effect, is negative; and as we approach the Y axis, the denominator approaches -0. Thus, in Fig. 8.11, as we move to the right along the arc from what we have identified as the lower limit in the lower left quadrant to the Y axis that bounds this quadrant on the right (a), our interval includes all of the ratios from 245,200 to $+\infty$.

   Alternatively, if we approach this same axis from the right in the lower right quadrant, we are approaching a cost-effectiveness ratio of $-\infty$. That is because the difference in cost is negative; the difference in effect is positive, and as we approach the Y axis, the denominator is approaching $+0$. Thus, as we move down along the arc from what we have identified as the upper limit in the upper right quadrant first to the X axis (b), which bounds this quadrant from below, our interval includes all of the ratios from 28,200 to 0. As we continue along the arc from the X axis that bounds the lower right quadrant from above to the Y axis that bounds this quadrant on the left (c), our interval also includes all of the ratios from 0 to $-\infty$.

   Thus, although the confidence interval for the cost-effectiveness ratio looks continuous on the cost-effectiveness plane, the interval includes the regions from 28,200 down to $-\infty$ and from 245,200 up to ∞, and it excludes a middle region between 28,200 and 245,200.

2. How is it possible for the lower limit to be a larger number than the upper limit?

   To help explain how the lower limit can be a larger number than the upper limit, in Fig. 8.12 we have superimposed a dashed line representing a cost-effectiveness ratio of 50,000 through the origin of the cost-effectiveness plane. A single line such as this through the origin represents the widest

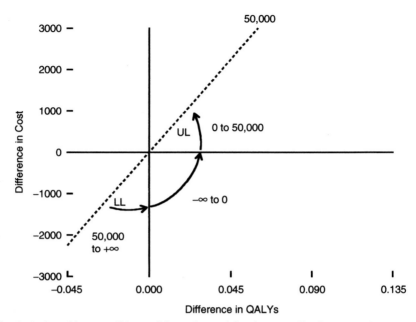

Fig. 8.12 The widest possible confidence interval for the cost-effectiveness ratio.

possible confidence interval for a cost-effectiveness ratio, because it includes all values of the ratio from −∞ to ∞ . As the current example is drawn, when the confidence interval includes the *Y* axis, the lower, clockwise, limit must be on or to the right of the dashed line on the left-hand side of the *Y* axis. As we have already explained, cost-effectiveness ratios in this region range from 50,000 to +∞ ; thus, the resulting limit must be greater than or equal to 50,000. At the same time, the upper, counterclockwise, limit must be on or below the dashed line on the right-hand side of the *Y* axis. If this limit falls in the upper right quadrant, it is a positive number that is less than or equal to 50,000; if it falls in the lower right quadrant, it is a negative number. Thus, when the confidence interval includes the *Y* axis, the lower clockwise limit must be a larger number than the upper counterclockwise limit.

This last explanation describes the technical geometric reasons how the lower limit can be greater than the upper limit, but does not help explain why the lower limit exceeds the upper limit. To better understand why this reversal occurs, recall that in Chapter 7 (pp. **135, 136**) we demonstrated that a ratio of the cost per unit of effect gained reports the trade-off of cost and effect for the therapy with the larger effect estimate in its denominator. In other words, if therapy A has a larger effect estimate in the denominator than therapy B, the resulting cost-effectiveness ratio will describe the extra cost for the extra effect of therapy A, independent of whether we subtract therapy B's estimates from therapy A's or vice versa.

When the confidence interval for effectiveness crosses the Y axis, the resulting interpretation is that therapy A may be more effective than therapy B or alternatively therapy B may be more effective than therapy A. For experiment 2, when we calculate the upper limit, we are working on the right side of the Y axis, which is the region of the distribution of the difference in cost and effect in which therapy A is more effective than therapy B. The resulting 28,200 upper limit indicates that we cannot rule out with 95% confidence that A is producing additional QALYs at a cost of up to 28,200 per QALY. When, on the other hand, we calculate the lower limit, we are working on the left side of the Y axis, which is the region of the distribution of the difference in cost and effect in which therapy B is more effective than A. The resulting 245,200 lower limit indicates we cannot rule out with 95% confidence that B is producing additional QALYs at a minimum cost of 245,200 per QALY.

Thus, for experiments like this one, the lower limit can – and indeed must – be greater than or equal to the upper limit, because each limit is describing the possible range of trade-offs between cost and effect for a different therapy. Therapy A may be more effective than therapy B, and if it is, we can be 95% confident that it's cost-effectiveness ratio falls in the range between $- \infty$ and 28,200. Alternatively, therapy B may be more effective than A, but if it is, we can be 95% confident that its cost-effectiveness ratio falls in the range between 245,200 and $+\infty$.

3. How is it possible that the point estimate is not bounded by the limits?

In experiment 2, the point estimate is 875; the lower limit is 245,200; and the upper limit is 28,200. The how and why that the point estimate is not bounded by the confidence limits is similar to the how and why of the relationship between the lower and upper limits. For the "How," in Fig. 8.12, the point estimate must fall below and to the right of both the lower and upper limits. If it falls in the lower left quadrant, it must be between the lower limit and the Y axis ($+\infty$), in which case the point estimate must be larger than the lower limit, and both are larger than the upper limit. If it falls in either the upper or lower right quadrants, it must be between the upper limit and the Y axis ($-\infty$), in which case it must be smaller than the upper limit, and both are smaller than the lower limit.

As to the why, the point estimate and one of the limits apply to the therapy with the larger point estimate for effect; the other limit applies to the therapy with the smaller point estimate for effect. In experiment 2, the point estimate falls on the right side of the Y axis, and the point estimate and the upper limit refer to the therapy A whereas the lower limit refers to therapy B. The fact that the point estimate is less than the upper limit makes sense in this case, because we typically want the upper limit to bound the point estimate from above. The reason the lower limit does not bound the point estimate from below is because this limit is no longer referring to therapy A, but instead is referring to therapy B.

If, on the other hand, the limits were the same, but the point estimate had fallen in the lower left quadrant, the fact that the lower limit would bound the point estimate from below again would make sense, because both the lower limit and the point estimate would be referring to therapy B. As with the prior example, the reason the upper limit would not bound the point estimate from above is because this limit would no longer be referring to therapy B, but instead would be referring to therapy A.

We began the discussion of experiment 2 by posing a challenge for cost-effectiveness ratios: given that the same confidence limits can describe two very different kinds of experiments – one where the effect estimate is significant and one where it is not – how do confidence intervals for cost-effectiveness ratios communicate which of the two experiments we are observing? The answer to this question is that they do so by reversing the confidence limits that define the interval. In other words, when we use the methods that we used to calculate the lower limit in experiment 1, we now derive a limit of 245,200 rather than 28,200. When we use the methods that we used to calculate the upper limit in experiment 1, we now derive a limit of 28,200 rather than 245,200. It would be a mistake to think that we can solve this inconsistency by simply switching the numbers and reporting a confidence interval that ranges from 28,200 to 245,200. That is the interval for an experiment like #1, in which the difference in effect is significant. When we see an interval in which the lower limit is greater than the upper limit, we know we are observing an experiment in which the difference in effect is not significant.

Finally, while the magnitude of experiment 2's confidence limits may or may not still be counterintuitive, these oddities do not change our methods for deriving confidence statements from confidence intervals for cost-effectiveness ratios. As with results like those in experiment 1, if our maximum willingness to pay falls within the confidence interval, we cannot be confident that the two therapies differ in their cost effectiveness. If, on the other hand, our maximum willingness to pay falls outside the interval, we can be 95% confident that one of the therapies is cost effective compared with the other. Thus, for experiment 2 if our maximum willingness to pay is between 28,200 and 245,200, we can be 95% confident that therapy A is good value compared to therapy B. If our maximum willingness to pay is less than 28,200 or greater than 245,200, we cannot be 95% confident that the economic value of A and B differs.

The fact that confidence intervals for cost-effectiveness ratios like those in experiment 2 are readily interpretable does not necessarily mean that more general audiences will always understand them. You yourself may still be bothered when we report in experiment 2 that the point estimate is 875 and that the lower and upper confidence limits are 245,200 and 28,200, respectively. We thus recommend that for experiments with this pattern of results, consider eliminating direct reporting of the confidence limits. Instead, consider reporting something like the following: we can be 95% confident that therapy A is cost-effective compared to therapy B if our willingness to pay is between 28,200 and 245,200 (i.e., 30,000 or 50,000); we cannot be 95% confident that the economic value of therapies A and B differs if our willingness to pay is less than 28,200 or greater than 245,200.

8.5.2. Confidence intervals for net monetary benefit (NMB) and acceptability curves

As we have indicated earlier, the challenge of communicating which of the two types of experiments we are observing is not limited to confidence intervals for cost-effectiveness ratios alone. It is also shared by confidence intervals for NMB and acceptability curves. Yes, for both experiments the NMB graphs have intersections between the NMB limits and the X axis at 28,200 and 245,200. But as we have already shown, in experiment 1 (and all other pattern 1 results), both the lower and the upper limits intersect this axis once. When evaluating confidence intervals for NMB, we know we are observing an experiment like experiment 2, in which the difference in effect is not significant, because one (in this case the lower) limit intersects the X axis twice and the other limit never intersects the X axis (see Fig. 8.13A).

Similarly, the acceptability curves both of experiments 1 and 2 cross the decision thresholds twice at 28,200 and/or 245,200. But as we have already shown, in experiment 1 as well as in other pattern 1 results, the acceptability curve intersects the horizontal lines at both 0.025 and 0.975. We know we are observing an experiment like experiment 2, however, when the acceptability curve intersects the horizontal line at either 0.025 or (in this case) 0.975 twice, and never intersects the other horizontal line (see Fig. 8.13B).

As with confidence intervals for cost-effectiveness ratios, the fact that only one of the NMB limits intersects the X axis twice and the fact that the acceptability curve does not intersect both 0.025 and 0.975 does not affect how we derive confidence statements from NMB graphs and acceptability curves.

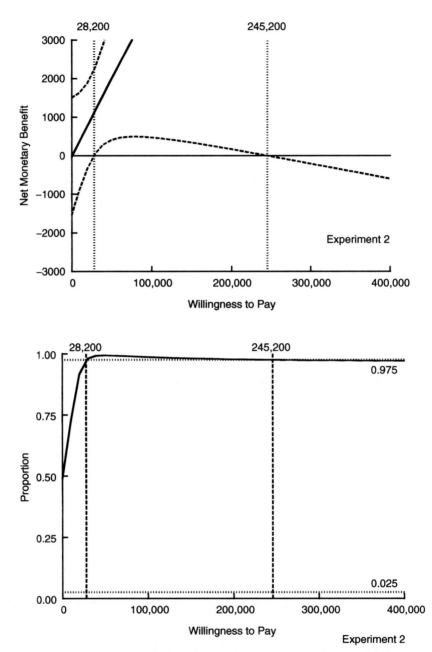

Fig. 8.13 Net monetary benefit (NMB) graph (A) and acceptability curve (B) for experiment 2.

For both experiments 1 and 2, when both NMB limits are above the X axis or when the acceptability curve is above 0.975, we can be confident that therapy A is good value compared with therapy B. Thus, as we found with the confidence intervals for the cost-effectiveness ratio, for willingnesses to pay between 28,200 and 245,200, we can be 95% confident that therapy A is cost-effective compared with therapy B. When both NMB limits are below the X axis or when the acceptability curve is below 0.025, we can be confident that therapy A is not good value compared with therapy B. Finally, when one of the NMB limits is positive and one negative or when the acceptability curve is between 0.025 and 0.975 (i.e., for maximum willingnesses to pay less than 28,200 or greater than 245,200), we cannot be confident that the two therapies are different.

8.5.3. Summary of findings for experiment 2

We refer to findings like those in experiment 2 as pattern 2 findings. Pattern 2 findings occur only when the difference in effect is not significant ($p > \alpha$ for effect when we are seeking $1 - \alpha$ confidence for determination of value for the cost), but it is not the only pattern of findings that can occur when the difference in effect is not significant (see experiment 3, below). We know we are observing a pattern 2 finding when the confidence interval for the cost-effectiveness ratio includes the Y axis, in which case the lower limit is greater than the upper limit and the point estimate is either greater than or less than both limits. We also know we are observing this pattern of findings when one NMB confidence limit crosses the decision threshold twice and when the acceptability curve intersects a horizontal line at either 0.025 or 0.975 twice and does not intersect the other horizontal line even once.

As shown in Fig. 8.14, when pattern 2 findings are defined over the range of willingnesses to pay from $-\infty$ to $+\infty$ they – like pattern 1 findings – are characterized by three ranges of willingness to pay for a unit of health outcome. The order of the ranges for the two patterns, however, differs. For pattern 2 experiments,

PATTERN #2

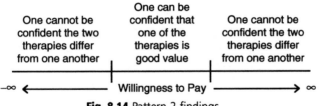

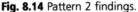

Fig. 8.14 Pattern 2 findings.

on both the left and the right are those values of willingness to pay for which we cannot be confident that the therapies differ. In the middle are those values of willingness to pay for which we can be confident that one therapy is good value compared with the other. In experiment 2, the boundaries between these ranges occur at 28,200 and 245,200.

Pattern 2 findings do not share the advantage of pattern 1 findings that if we are confident that the more effective therapy is good value at a specific willingness to pay, we can be confident that it will be good value for all larger willingnesses to pay and if we are confident that it is not good value at a specific willingness to pay, we can be confident that it will not be good value for all smaller willingnesses to pay. Instead, for pattern 2, if we are confident that one therapy is good value compared to the other, we know that there are both higher and lower willingnesses to pay for which we cannot be confident about its value. Thus, for experiments with this pattern of results, precise knowledge about our maximum willingness to pay for a unit of health outcome may be more important than it is for experiments that have pattern 1 results.

As with pattern 1, observation of pattern 2 findings is independent of the method we use to address sampling uncertainty. The three ranges of willingness to pay that are observed for pattern 2 findings are defined identically by the confidence interval for the cost-effectiveness ratio, the confidence interval for NMB, and the acceptability curve. As with pattern 1, observation of a pattern 2 finding depends upon the data as well as the level of confidence we desire. For example, except for certain experiments that have a point estimate for effect of 0, all experiments that demonstrate pattern 2 findings for statements of 95% confidence will demonstrate pattern 1 findings for some (possibly extremely) lower levels of confidence.

Finally, as with pattern 1, left and right truncation can mask the pattern we are observing on the NMB graph and the acceptability curves, but such uncertainty never arises for confidence intervals for cost-effectiveness ratios.

8.6. **Experiment 3, another unfamiliar pattern of results**

Suppose you conducted an economic evaluation of two therapies and found that therapy A on average cost 400 more than therapy B (SE, 325, p = 0.22); therapy A on average yielded 0.02 QALYs more than therapy B (SE, 0.02, p = 0.32); the correlation between the difference in cost and effect was 0.25; and there were 250 participants per group in the trial.

The point estimate of the cost-effectiveness ratio for this experiment is 20,000 (400/0.02). Inspection of Fig. 8.15A suggests that it is impossible to

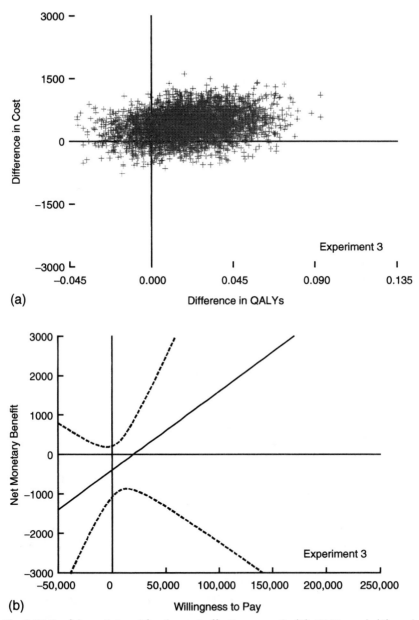

(a)

(b)

Fig. 8.15 Confidence interval for the cost-effectiveness ratio (A), NMB graph (A), and the acceptability curve (B) for experiment 3.

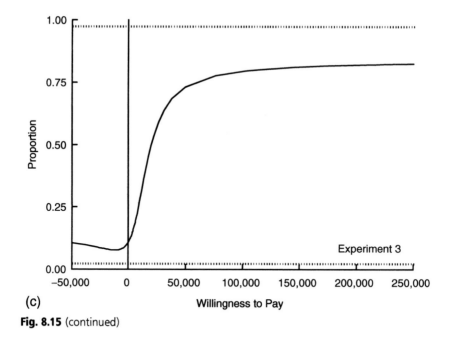

(c)

Fig. 8.15 (continued)

draw a line through the origin that excludes 2.5% of the distribution of the difference in cost and effect, which means that the confidence interval for the cost-effectiveness ratio cannot be defined. In fact, the smallest fraction of the distribution of the difference that can be excluded by a line through the origin is 7.76% (cost-effectiveness ratio, −11,500), in which case the largest definable confidence interval for the cost-effectiveness ratio is the 84.48% $(1 - (2 \times 0.0776))$ interval. Given that we can be 95% confident that the two therapies differ only if our maximum willingness to pay is excluded by the experiment's confidence interval for the cost-effectiveness ratio, and given that when the confidence interval for the cost-effectiveness ratio is undefined, it cannot exclude any willingness to pay, for this experiment, there is no willingness to pay for which we can be 95% confident that the economic value of therapies A and B differs from one another.

When it is impossible to define a 95% confidence interval for the cost-effectiveness ratio, then neither of the 95% confidence limits for NMB intersect the X axis (see Fig. 8.15B), and thus for all willingnesses to pay, the NMB confidence interval must include 0. Similarly, when it is impossible to define a 95% confidence interval for the cost-effectiveness ratio, the acceptability curve never intersects the horizontal lines drawn at 0.025 and 0.975 on the Y axis (see Fig. 8.15C). Thus, the confidence interval for NMB and the acceptability curve confirms the conclusion we derive from the fact that no confidence interval for the cost-effectiveness ratio can be defined: there is no willingness to pay for which we can be confident that the economic value of therapies A and B differs from one another.

8.6.1. Summary of findings for experiment 3

We refer to findings like those in experiment 3 as pattern 3 findings. As with pattern 2, pattern 3 findings occur only when the difference in effect is not significant. We know we are observing a pattern 3 finding when the confidence interval for the cost-effectiveness ratio is undefined, when the NMB limits never intersect the X axis, and when the acceptability curve fails to intersect horizontal lines drawn at 0.025 and 0.975.

As shown in Fig. 8.16, unlike patterns 1 and 2, pattern 3 findings are characterized by a single range of willingness to pay for a unit of health outcome, the range where we cannot be confident that the two therapies differ from one another.

As with patterns 1 and 2, observation of pattern 3 findings is independent of the method we use to address sampling uncertainty: all three methods for addressing sampling uncertainty indicate a lack of 95% confidence that the therapies differ. As with patterns 1 and 2, observation of a pattern 3 finding depends upon the data as well as the level of confidence we desire. For example, except for some special cases, all experiments that demonstrate pattern 3 findings for statements of 95% confidence will demonstrate pattern 1 and pattern 2 findings for some (possibly extremely) lower levels of confidence.

Finally, as with patterns 1 and 2, left and right truncation may mask the pattern we are observing on the NMB graph and the acceptability curves, but such uncertainty never arises for confidence intervals for cost-effectiveness ratios.

8.7. Conclusions from the three experiments

The three experiments represent examples of the three distinct patterns of results we can observe when we compare therapies' value for the cost (see Fig. 8.17). Pattern 1 has three ranges of willingness to pay. From left to

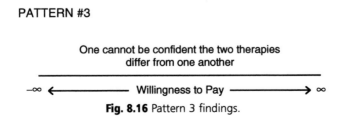

PATTERN #3

One cannot be confident the two therapies
differ from one another

$-\infty$ ⟵ ——————— Willingness to Pay ——————— ⟶ ∞

Fig. 8.16 Pattern 3 findings.

right they represent willingnesses to pay for which we can be confident that the therapy with the larger point estimate for effect is not good value, willingnesses to pay for which we cannot be confident that the economic value of the two therapies' differs, and willingnesses to pay for which we can be confident that the therapy with the larger point estimate for effect is good value. Pattern 2 experiments also have three ranges of willingness to pay. From left to right they represent willingnesses to pay for which we cannot be confident that the economic value of the two therapies' differs, willingnesses to pay for which we can be confident that the therapy with the larger point estimate for effect is good value, and again willingnesses to pay for which we cannot be confident that the economic value of the two therapies' differs. Pattern 3 has one range of willingness to pay in which we cannot be confident that the value for the cost of the two therapies differs.

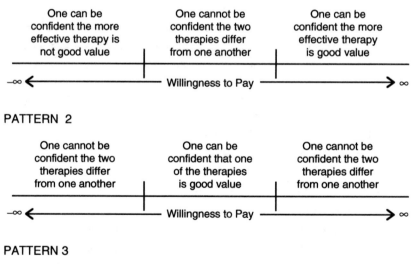

PATTERN 1

| One can be confident the more effective therapy is not good value | One cannot be confident the two therapies differ from one another | One can be confident the more effective therapy is good value |

−∞ ← ——————————— Willingness to Pay ——————————— → ∞

PATTERN 2

| One cannot be confident the two therapies differ from one another | One can be confident that one of the therapies is good value | One cannot be confident the two therapies differ from one another |

−∞ ← ——————————— Willingness to Pay ——————————— → ∞

PATTERN 3

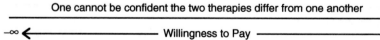

One cannot be confident the two therapies differ from one another

−∞ ← ——————————— Willingness to Pay ——————————— → ∞

Fig. 8.17 Summary of three patterns of results for the comparison of two strategies. The pattern that is observed is independent of whether we use cost-effectiveness ratios, net monetary benefit (NMB), or acceptability curves to express differences in value between strategies. More effective is the strategy with the larger point estimate for effectiveness.

Confidence intervals for cost-effectiveness ratios, NMB, and acceptability curves can all be used to address sampling uncertainty related to determination of value for the cost. No matter which of the three patterns of results we observe, all three methods for addressing sampling uncertainty yield the same conclusions about confidence. In other words, if one method indicates that we can be confident that therapy A is good value compared with therapy B, the other two methods will also indicate we can be confident of therapy A's value. If one method indicates we cannot be confident, then the other two will also indicate we cannot be confident.

The boundaries between ranges of willingness to pay for units of health outcome where we can or cannot be confident are identified by the confidence interval for the cost-effectiveness ratio. Thus, if our primary goal is to inform our audience about the willingness to pay for which they can and cannot be confident about a therapy's value for the cost, these limits provide the necessary information. Even when the resulting confidence intervals have odd properties, they provide this information. For example, if the confidence interval for the cost-effectiveness ratio is undefined, it means there is no willingness to pay for which we can be confident that the economic value of therapy A differs from that of therapy B.

The boundaries between ranges of willingness to pay can be identical for two very different experiments. In one experiment, the difference in effect is significant and the confidence interval for the cost-effectiveness ratio excludes the Y axis of the cost-effectiveness plane. In the other, the difference in effect is insignificant and the confidence interval for the cost-effectiveness ratio includes the Y axis. In one experiment the difference in cost is significant, whereas in the other experiment it is not. Finally, in one we can be confident about value for the cost, whereas in the other we cannot be confident. As indicated in Fig. 8.17, in instances where these different experiments share the same boundaries, what differs is the ordering of the confidence ranges between the boundaries.

All three methods do something unexpected to communicate which type of experiment, and thus which ordering of confidence ranges, is being observed. The lower confidence limit for the cost-effectiveness ratio is smaller than the upper limit for a pattern 1 result, whereas the limits are reversed (i.e., lower limit larger than the upper limit) when a pattern 2 result is observed. Both NMB limits intersect the X axis when we observe a pattern 1 result, whereas one of the limits intersects the X axis twice and the other limit never intersects this axis when we observe a pattern 2 result. Finally, the acceptability curve intersects horizontal lines at 0.025 and 0.975 when we observe a pattern 1 result, whereas it intersects either the line at 0.025 or the line at 0.975 twice

Table 8.1. Cues for identifying patterns

Pattern	Method		
	Cost-effectiveness ratio	Net monetary benefit (NMB)	Acceptability curve
1	The lower confidence limit is less than the upper confidence limit and the point estimate is between the two limits.	Each of the two confidence limits intersect the X axis once and only once.	The acceptability curve intersects each of the decision thresholds once and only once, and the curve increases monotonically between the decision thresholds
2	The lower confidence limit is greater than the upper confidence limit, and the point estimate is greater or smaller than both limits.	One confidence limit intersects the X axis twice, and the other confidence limit does not intersect the X axis at all.	The acceptability curve intersects one of the decision thresholds twice and does not intersect the other decision threshold.
3	The confidence interval is undefined.	Neither confidence limit intersects or is tangent to the X axis.	The acceptability curve never intersects or is tangent to the decision thresholds.

and never intersects the other line when we observe a pattern 2 result. See Table 8.1 for a summary of the cues for identifying the three patterns.

Finally, if we want to vary one's confidence level, for confidence intervals for cost-effectiveness ratios and confidence intervals for NMB, we need to calculate additional sets of confidence intervals (e.g., 75 or 90% intervals). As shown in Fig. 8.7, the acceptability curve has the advantage that it reports confidence intervals for cost-effectiveness ratios – and thus boundaries between confidence ranges – for varying levels of confidence.

References

1. O'Brien BJ, Drummond MF, Labelle RJ, Willan A. In search of power and significance: issues in the design and analysis of stochastic cost-effectiveness studies in health care. *Med Care* 1994; 32: 150–63.
2. Glick HA, Briggs AH, Polsky D. Quantifying stochastic uncertainty and presenting the results of cost effectiveness analyses. *Expert Rev Pharmacoeconomics Outcomes Res*. 2001; 1: 25–36.
3. Willan A, Lin DY. Incremental net benefit in randomized controlled trials. *Stat Med*. 2001; 20: 1563–74.
4. Heitjan DF. Fieller's method and net health benefits. *Health Econ*. 2000; 9: 327–35.
5. van Hout BA, Al MJ, Gordon GS, Rutten FFH. Costs, effects, and C/E ratios alongside a clinical trial. *Health Econ*. 1994; 3: 309–19.

6. Briggs A, Fenn P. Confidence intervals or surfaces? Uncertainty on the cost-effectiveness plane. *Health Econ.* 1998; 7: 723–40.

7. Lothgren M, Zethraeus N. Definition, interpretation and calculation of cost-effectiveness acceptability curves. *Health Econ.* 2000; 9: 623–30.

8. Fenwick E, O'Brien BJ, Briggs A, Cost-effectiveness acceptability curves – facts, fallacies and frequently asked questions. *Health Econ.* 2004; 13: 405–15.

Chapter 9

Sampling uncertainty: calculation, sample size and power, and decision criteria

In Chapter 8, we demonstrated the quantification and interpretation of sampling uncertainty by use of confidence intervals for cost-effectiveness ratios, confidence intervals for NMB, and acceptability curves; we also identified and interpreted hard cases. In doing so, we identified three distinct patterns of results into which all experiments fall. In this chapter, we introduce methods of calculation, identify when the three patterns of experiments are observed; provide methods for calculation of sample size and power for evaluation of economic outcomes; and describe revisions to decision rules for choosing therapies that are prompted by consideration of sampling uncertainty.

9.1. Calculating confidence intervals for cost-effectiveness ratios

Confidence intervals for cost-effectiveness ratios provide a probabilistic range of values within which we can be confident that the true cost-effectiveness ratio lies. As with confidence intervals for NMB and acceptability curves, confidence intervals for cost-effectiveness ratios can be constructed by use of parametric methods or nonparametric ones, the latter by use of a bootstrap procedure. When parametric methods are used to estimate this uncertainty, all three methods for quantifying sampling uncertainty assume that the difference in cost and effect is distributed bivariate normal. Dependably accurate parametric confidence intervals for cost-effectiveness ratios can be derived by use of Fieller's method [1–5].

9.1.1. Fieller's method

This parametric method is based on the assumption that the expression $RQ - C$ is normally distributed with mean zero, where R equals C/Q, Q equals the difference in arithmetic mean effect, and C equals the difference in arithmetic mean cost. Standardizing this statistic by its standard error and setting it equal to the critical value from a Student's t distribution generates a quadratic equation in R. The roots of this equation give the confidence limits:

$$\text{CER}_{CL} =$$

$$\frac{(CQ - t_{\alpha/2}^2 \rho se_c se_q) \pm \left\{ (CQ - t_{\alpha/2}^2 \rho se_c se_q)^2 - (Q^2 - t_{\alpha/2}^2 se_q^2)(C^2 - t_{\alpha/2}^2 se_c^2) \right\}^{0.5}}{Q^2 - t_{\alpha/2}^2 se_q^2}, \quad (9.1)$$

where CER_{CL} is the $1-\alpha$ confidence limit for the cost-effectiveness ratio; $t_{\alpha/2}$ is the t statistic representing the decision makers' desired two-tailed level of confidence; ρ is the correlation between the difference in cost and effect; and se_c and se_q are the standard errors for the difference in cost and effect, respectively. Independent of the magnitude of the resulting limits, the lower, or clockwise, limit is derived by subtracting the term on right-hand side of the numerator from the term on the left-hand side; the upper, or counterclockwise, limit is derived by adding these two terms.

To the equation phobic, this equation may look unsettling. Before being frightened off, however, you should note that it is comprised of three basic equations, two of which are repeated twice. One of these equations is made up of cost, its standard error, and a t value that represents the desired level of confidence. It appears once at the far right of the numerator of the confidence limit equation.

$$C^2 - t_{\alpha/2}^2 se_c^2$$

A second equation has the same structure as the cost equation above, but substitutes the difference in effect, its standard error, and a t value. It appears just to the left of the cost equation in the numerator and in the denominator of the confidence limit equation.

$$Q^2 - t_{\alpha/2}^2 se_q^2$$

The third is made up of cost and effect, their standard errors, a t value, and the correlation of the difference in cost and effect. It appears twice on the left side of the numerator of the confidence limit equation.

$$CQ - t_{\alpha/2}^2 \rho se_c se_q$$

In fact, to avoid programming errors, in our programs for this equation we calculate the results of each of these three equations separately and then combine them into the confidence limit equation.

As with experiment 3 in Chapter 8, when there is no line through the origin that can exclude α/2% of the distribution of the difference in cost and effect, the resulting limits from this equation are undefined.

The data needed to calculate these limits can be obtained from common statistical packages by testing the difference in cost and obtaining C and se_c, testing the difference in effect and obtaining Q and se_q, and estimating the Pearson correlation between the difference in cost and effect (see Box 9.1 for its derivation). These variables, along with the t statistic, are then combined to derive the Fieller's method interval.

9.1.2. **Nonparametric bootstrap methods**

As we indicated in Chapter 5, bootstrap methods are based on generating multiple replications of the statistic of interest by sampling with replacement from the original data [6]. A number of bootstrap methods are available for constructing confidence intervals for cost-effectiveness ratios. The most common nonparametric method used in the literature is the bootstrap percentile method [4,7]. This method is dependably accurate when the difference in effect is statistically significant (pattern 1 finding); however it can fail in its accuracy when the difference in effect is not significant. Alternatively, one can use what we refer to as the nonparametric acceptability method. This method calculates confidence limits by identifying lines through the origin that omit α/2 of the distribution of the difference in cost and effect, and – like Fieller's method intervals – is dependably accurate independent of the pattern of experiment that is observed.

Bootstrap percentile method

As we indicated in Chapter 5, by this method, we derive a confidence interval by repeatedly drawing samples with replacement from the original treatment arms in the study and using the resulting data to compute bootstrap replications of the statistic of interest, in this case, the cost-effectiveness ratio. By convention, at least 1000 bootstrap replications are constructed [6]. We define the confidence limits by next ordering the replications of the ratio from lowest to highest or best to worst, being sure to distinguish replicates whose ratios have the same sign, but which fall in different quadrants of the cost-effectiveness plane. Finally, we determine the limits by identifying the ratios from the replicates that bound the α/2 and $1-(\alpha$/2) percentiles of the distribution of the difference in cost and effect. For example, if there are 1000 bootstrap replicates, and if we wish to construct 95% confidence limits, they are defined by the ratios for the 26th and 975th ordered replicates; if there are 2000 replicates, they are defined by the ratios for the 51st and 1950th ordered replicates.

Box 9.1 Calculation of the correlation of the difference

The correlation between the difference in cost and effect is derived from the joint variance of cost, the joint variance of effect, and the joint covariance of cost and effect. The joint variance of cost is calculated by taking the weighted average of the variance of cost in treatment groups 0 (CV_0) and 1 (CV_1), with weights based on the number of participants in each arm of the trial:

$$JCV = \frac{(N_0 - 1)CV_0 + (N_1 - 1)CV_1}{N_0 + N_1 - 2}$$

The joint variance of effect is calculated by taking the weighted average of the variance of effect in treatment groups 0 (QV_0) and 1 (QV_1):

$$JQV = \frac{(N_0 - 1)QV_0 + (N_1 - 1)QV_1}{N_0 + N_1 - 2}$$

The joint covariance of cost and effect is calculated by taking the weighted average of the covariance of cost and effect in treatment groups 0 (Cov_0) and 1 (Cov_1):

$$JCOV = \frac{(N_0 - 1)Cov_0 + (N_1 - 1)Cov_1}{N_0 + N_1 - 2}$$

Finally, the correlation of the difference in cost and effect that is used to estimate Fieller's method confidence intervals, parametric confidence intervals for NMB, and the parametric acceptability curve is calculated by dividing the joint covariance of cost and effect by the product of the square roots of the joint variances of cost and effect.

$$\rho = \frac{JCOV}{JCV^{0.5} \times JQV^{0.5}}$$

Ordering is complicated when an experiment's joint distribution of the difference in cost and effect has nonnegligible amounts of its density in all four quadrants of the cost-effectiveness plane. Although there is no consensus in the literature, by use of simulation we have found that the resulting limits are most like the Fieller's and bootstrap acceptability methods' results if the replicates are ranked counterclockwise lexicographically by quadrant and by ratio. As shown in Fig. 9.1, the ordering begins in the quadrant opposite to that in which the point estimate lies, rotates counterclockwise for 360°, and returns to the quadrant opposite to that in which the point estimate lies.

Bootstrap acceptability method

As with the percentile method confidence interval, the bootstrap acceptability method confidence interval is derived by repeatedly drawing samples with replacement from the original treatment arms in the study and using the resulting data to compute bootstrap replications of the difference in cost and effect and the cost-effectiveness ratio. The difference between the two methods arises only after computation of these replications. We use each of the resulting bootstrap replications of the cost-effectiveness ratio to define the slope of a line through the origin of the cost-effectiveness plane, and construct 1-α % confidence intervals by identifying the slopes for those lines that exclude α /2% of the bootstrap replicates. This method is referred to as the acceptability method, because – except for the fact that we evaluate both negative and positive ratios – we construct the interval by use of a method identical to that used to construct a bootstrap acceptability curve (see p. **185**, below).

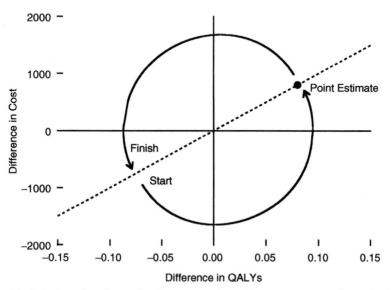

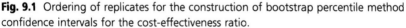

Fig. 9.1 Ordering of replicates for the construction of bootstrap percentile method confidence intervals for the cost-effectiveness ratio.

The fact that the percentile method's confidence interval may not always be dependably accurate does not mean we should reject use of this computationally less intensive method outright in favor of the acceptability method. It can be shown that the percentile method interval is dependably accurate when each of its limits – when defined as a line through the origin – excludes approximately $\alpha/2\%$ of the distribution of the difference in cost and effect, and fails in its accuracy when each of its limits – when defined as a line through the origin – excludes substantially more than $\alpha/2\%$. Such failures generally occur when there is a non-negligible proportion of the distribution of the difference in cost and effect that is simultaneously excluded by both limits, which usually does not occur when the difference in effect is significant. Thus, after construction of percentile method limits, investigators can evaluate the fraction of the distribution of the difference in cost and effect that is excluded by each limit – when defined as a line through the origin – and judge whether the resulting interval is likely to be accurate.

9.2. Calculating confidence intervals for net monetary benefit (NMB)

Unlike the cost-effectiveness ratio, whose distribution can suffer discontinuities and for which the variance is not always defined, net monetary benefit (NMB) is continuous, and its variance, and thus its standard error, is well defined. The standard error for NMB equals:

$$SE_{NMB} = (se_c^2 + W^2 se_q^2 - 2W\rho se_c se_q)^{0.5}, \qquad (9.2)$$

where W equals the willingness to pay. The formula for the confidence interval for NMB equals:

$$NMB_{CL} = (WQ - C) \pm t_{\alpha/2}(se_c^2 + W^2 se_q^2 - 2W\rho se_c se_q)^{0.5}, \qquad (9.3)$$

You will note that except for the term W, we use the same information to calculate confidence intervals for NMB that we did to calculate confidence intervals for cost-effectiveness ratios: difference in cost and its standard error; difference in effect and its standard error; correlation of the difference in cost and effect; and the t statistic representing the decision makers' desired level of confidence. Unlike confidence intervals for cost-effectiveness ratios, the smaller NMB limit is always the lower limit.

The confidence interval for NMB can also be calculated nonparametrically. As with bootstrapped confidence intervals for cost-effectiveness ratios, we derive the interval by repeatedly drawing samples with replacement from the original treatment arms in the study and using the resulting data to compute bootstrap replications of NMB. As with the bootstrap percentile method, we define the confidence limits by ordering the replications of NMB from lowest to highest and identifying the NMBs from the replicates that bound the $\alpha/2$ and $1-(\alpha/2)$ percentiles of the distribution of NMB.

9.3. Calculating acceptability curves

Acceptability curves can be constructed parametrically by solving for Fieller's method limits for varying levels of confidence, i.e., for a range of values for $t_{\alpha/2}$. We can also derive them parametrically by varying levels of the willingness to pay, and solving for the t statistic where the NMB confidence limit equals 0. The latter formula equals:

$$t_{\alpha/2} = \sqrt{\frac{(WQ-C)^2}{se_c^2 + Wse_q^2 - 2W\rho se_c se_q}} \tag{9.4}$$

When constructing the acceptability curve for the strategy with the larger point estimate for effectiveness – i.e., the more effective strategy – when W is less than the point estimate for the cost-effectiveness ratio, the height of the acceptability curve equals the proportion of the tail that is excluded at $t_{\alpha/2}$ (e.g., in Stata®, ttail(dof,$t_{\alpha/2}$)). When the willingness to pay is greater than the point estimate for the cost-effectiveness ratio, the height of the acceptability curve equals 1 minus the proportion of the tail that is excluded by the resulting $t_{\alpha/2}$ (e.g., in Stata®, 1–ttail(dof,$t_{\alpha/2}$)).

The acceptability curve can also be constructed nonparametrically by calculation of the proportion of bootstrap replicates falling on the acceptable side of the line through the origin that represents the willingness to pay. In Fig. 9.2, this method is applied to bootstrap data that were derived from experiment 1 in Chapter 8. Common features of the acceptability curve are described in Box 9.2 (p. 187).

9.4. Identifying the better-valued therapy

Table 9.1 (p. 189) reports relationships between cost-effectiveness ratios' and NMBs' point estimates, confidence limits, and decision criteria and the resulting confidence statements they support. It also reports relationships between the acceptability curve and decision criteria and the resulting confidence statements they support. For NMB, the confidence statements depend on whether the maximum willingness to pay falls inside or outside the confidence interval. For the acceptability curve, they depend on whether the curve is above, below, or between 0.025 and 0.975.

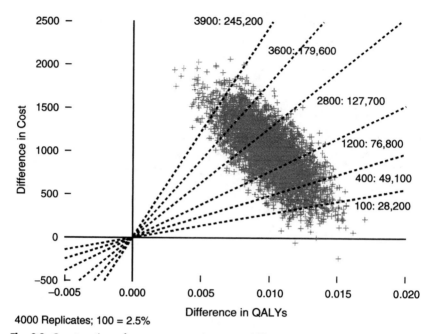

Fig. 9.2 Construction of a nonparametric acceptability curve.

As with NMB, confidence statements derived from confidence intervals for cost-effectiveness ratios depend on whether the maximum willingness to pay falls inside or outside the confidence interval. If the maximum willingness to pay falls within the interval, we cannot be confident that the therapies differ. If it falls outside the interval, and if the point estimate for the cost-effectiveness ratio is less than the maximum willingness to pay, we can be confident that the therapy with the larger point estimate for effect represents good value. If it falls outside the interval, and if the point estimate for the cost-effectiveness ratio is greater than the maximum willingness to pay, we can be confident that the therapy with the smaller point estimate for effect represents good value.

The one case where the logic underlying this relationship may be less clear is for the middle range of pattern 2 results in which our maximum willingness to pay falls outside the confidence interval. We have said earlier that this middle range of results indicates we can be 95% confident that one therapy is better value than another. We have not, however, given detailed information about the relationships between the point estimate, confidence limits, and maximum willingness to pay that indicate that the therapy with the larger point estimate for effectiveness is good or bad value.

Box 9.2 Geometry of the acceptability curve

Except for one class of unimodal distributions (discussed below), if we define the acceptability curve for values of willingness to pay for health ranging from $-\infty$ to $+\infty$, it will always have a common set of features. First, the curve will always have a section that is concave and monotonically changing, i.e., concave up or down and monotonically increasing or decreasing; see solid line, Fig. B9.1.1. Second, it will also always have a section that looks like a skewed distribution, i.e., skewed left or right; see dashed line, particularly the inset, Fig. B9.1.1.

As the willingness to pay approaches $-\infty$, the curve asymptotically approaches the proportion of the distribution of the difference in effect that is less than (greater than) 0 (see point A, Fig B9.1.1). As the willingness to pay approaches ∞, the curve asymptotically approaches the proportion of the distribution of the difference in effect that is greater than (less than) 0 (see point B, Fig. B9.1.1).

If we assume that the difference in cost and effect is bivariate normal, and construct a parametric acceptability curve, the boundaries between these different regions are defined by the formula for Fieller's theorem confidence limits. The concave, monotonically increasing section is defined over the range of values of willingness to pay for which the denominator of the Fieller's theorem formula is positive. In this region, the acceptability curve crosses both p and $1-p$ once and only once. All these results represent pattern 1 findings.

The skewed left (right) section is defined over the range of values of willingness to pay for which the denominator of the Fieller's theorem formula is negative and the rooted term in the numerator is nonnegative. All these results represent pattern 2. In this region, except in one instance, the acceptability curve crosses p (or $1-p$) twice and never crosses $1-p$ (or p). For example, if it crosses 0.10 twice, it never crosses 0.9.

The one instance where the acceptability curve does not cross p or $1-p$ twice is defined by the willingness to pay value where the rooted term in the numerator of the Fieller's theorem formula equals 0. In this case, the Fieller's theorem lower and upper confidence limits are equal, and the acceptability curve is tangent with p or $1-p$ once and only once (see point c, Fig. B9.1.1, which reaches a minimum of 0.012784 when the willingness to pay equals -5000). The acceptability curve never goes below this value of p (above $1-p$). This minimum (maximum) defines the boundary between

---

Box 9.2 Geometry of the acceptability curve *(continued)*

patterns 2 and 3. If we require more confidence than this level of p to choose a therapy, we simply do not have sufficient evidence to do so.

There is one class of unimodal distributions that does not share this pattern of acceptability curves. Centric distributions, which are symmetric over the origin, have acceptability curves that are horizontal at $p = 0.50$.

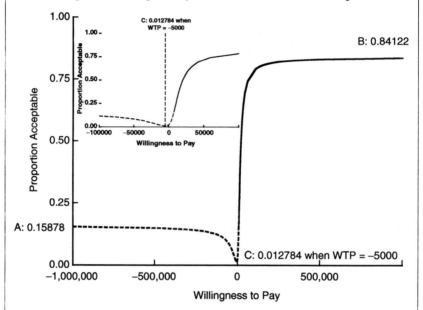

Fig. B9.1.1 Parametric acceptability curve for a distribution characterized by a difference in cost that equals 1000 (SE = 500), a difference in effect of 0.05 (SE = 0.05), a correlation of the difference in cost and effect of 0.0, and 1000 degrees of freedom. The curve has two regions, one that is concave and monotonically increasing (solid line) and one that is like a skewed distribution (dashed line). The inset, which magnifies the region of the curve between −100,000 and 100,000, shows that the apparent discontinuity at −5000 arises due to the scale of the figure.

Fig. 9.3 shows two pattern 2 experiments with the same confidence interval for the cost-effectiveness ratio, but with two different point estimates for this ratio. Experiment 2A is the same as experiment 2 in Chapter 8. If our maximum willingness to pay (e.g., 30,000 – 50,000) falls outside the interval, and if the point estimate for the cost-effectiveness ratio is smaller than the maximum willingness to pay, we conclude therapy A – which has the larger

Table 9.1 Confidence statements and the results that lead to them for patterns 1 and 2†

Confidence statement	Cost-effectiveness ratio	Net monetary benefit curve	Acceptability curve
Pattern 1	$(LL < PE < UL)$		
Can be 1−α confident that ME is good value	$LL < UL < W^*$	At W^*: $0 < LL < UL$	At W^*, curve is above 1−α/2
Cannot be 1−α confident that ME (or LE) is good value	$LL < W^* < UL$	At W^*: $LL < 0 < UL$	At W^*, curve is between α/2 and 1−α/2
Can be 1−α confident that ME is not good value	$W^* < LL < UL$	At W^*: $LL < UL < 0$	At W^*, curve is below α/2
Can be 1−α confident that ME statistically dominates LE	$LL < UL < 0$	When $W = 0$: $LL > 0$	When $W = 0$, curve is above 1−α/2
Pattern 2	$PE < UL < LL$ or $UL < LL < PE$		
Can be 1−α confident that ME is good value	$LL > W^* > UL > PE$	At W^*: $0 < LL < UL$	At W^*, curve is above 1−α/2
Cannot be 1−α confident that ME (or LE) is good value	$W^* > LL > UL$ or $LL > UL > W^*$	At W^*: $LL < 0 < UL$	At W^*, curve is between α/2 and 1−α/2
Can be 1−α confident that ME is not good value	$PE > LL > W^* > UL$	At W^*: $LL < UL < 0$	At W^*, curve is below α/2
Can be 1−α confident that ME statistically dominates LE	–	–	–

†PE is the point estimate for the cost-effectiveness ratio; ME is the strategy with the larger point estimate for effectiveness; LE is the strategy with the smaller point estimate for effectiveness; LL is the lower confidence limit; UL is the upper confidence limit; W^* is the maximum willingness to pay.

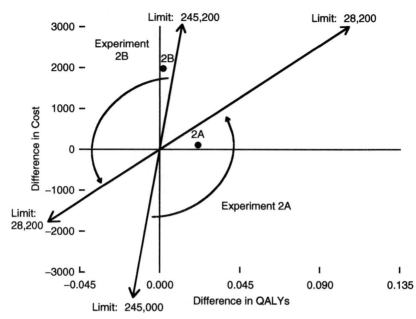

Fig. 9.3 Two pattern 2 experiments (2A and 2B). In experiment 2A, the point estimate indicates that therapy A is more costly and more effective than therapy B (the dot labeled 2A), and for willingnesses to pay ranging between 28,200 and 245,200 we can be 95% confident that it is good value compared to B. For all other willingnesses to pay, we cannot be confident that the two therapies differ. In experiment 2B, the point estimate indicates that therapy A continues to be more costly and more effective than therapy B (the dot labeled 2B), but we either can be confident that therapy A is not good value compared to therapy B (for willingnesses to pay between 28,200 and 245,200) or cannot be confident that the two therapies differ.

point estimate for effect – is good value. We do so because the confidence limits indicate that either it is more costly and more effective, in which case we are 95% confident that we will be spending at most 28,200 per QALY gained, or it is less costly and less effective, but we are 95% confident that we would need to spend at least 245,200 per QALY if we were to adopt therapy B.

Experiment 2B is a third experiment that along with experiments 1 and 2 share confidence limits that round to 28,200 and 245,200. Had you conducted this experiment, you might have found that therapy A on average cost 1985 more than therapy B (SE, 1252.1, p = 0.11); therapy A on average yielded 0.0001 QALYs more than therapy B (SE, 0.0089, p = 0.99); the correlation between the difference in cost and effect was 0.976; and there were 250 participants per group in the trial. Like experiment 2A, this experiment also falls into pattern 2, but differs from experiment 2A in that the point estimate (19,850,000 (1985/0.0001)) is greater than the lower limit, which is greater than the maximum willingness to pay, which finally is greater than the upper limit. For this experiment, we conclude that therapy A is not good value, because the point estimate for the cost-effectiveness ratio is larger than the maximum willingness to pay. The confidence limits indicate that either it is more costly and more effective, in which case we are 95% confident that we must spend at least 245,200 per QALY gained, or it is less costly and less effective, in which case we are 95% confident that the most we would need to spend is 28,200 per QALY gained if we were to adopt therapy B.

9.5. **When are the different patterns observed?**

If we are evaluating 95% confidence statements and we observe a pattern 1 result – for example, if the 95% confidence interval for the cost-effectiveness ratio is defined and its lower limit is less than the point estimate which in turn is less than its upper limit – there is no requirement that we will observe a pattern 1 result for all higher levels of confidence, for example 99%. Similarly, if we are evaluating 95% confidence statements and we observe a pattern 2 or 3 result – for example, if the 95% confidence interval for the cost-effectiveness ratio is undefined – that does not mean we will be unable to observe a pattern 1 result for a lower level of confidence, for example, 90%. Except for a few special cases, such as centric distributions that are symmetric over the origin, all distributions of the difference in cost and effect can be made to display all three patterns of results. They can be made to do so because the patterns are a function of the data and the level of confidence we wish to have. Thus, for example, if we cannot define a 95% confidence interval, one option is to identify a narrower interval that is definable.

Inspection of the formula for deriving Fieller's method confidence limits for the cost-effectiveness ratio (equation 9.1, p. **180**) indicates there are two situations where it is ill behaved. One occurs when the denominator equals 0, in which case the limits go to ∞. The other occurs when the rooted term in the numerator is negative (because we cannot take the square root of a negative number). These situations also mark the transitions between the three patterns of results. Pattern 2 results occur when the denominator is less than 0 and the rooted term in the numerator is greater than 0. Pattern 3 results occur when the rooted term in the numerator is negative.

We can simplify and rearrange the formula for Fieller's method confidence limits to determine the levels of confidence that fall into the three patterns. The boundary between patterns 1 and 2 is defined by the level of confidence associated with the t statistic that equals Q/se_q (derived by solving for the

t statistic that equates the denominator of eqn 9.1 to 0). In other words, for all levels of confidence associated with t statistics less than Q/se_q, we will observe a pattern 1 result.

The boundary between patterns 2 and 3 is defined by the level of confidence associated with the following t statistic:

$$t_{\alpha/2} = \sqrt{\frac{Q^2\left(\left[\dfrac{(C/Q)se_q - \rho se_c}{se_c}\right](1-\rho^2)\right)}{(1-\rho^2)se_q^2}} \qquad (9.5)$$

This equation was derived by solving for the t statistic that equates the rooted term in the numerator of eqn 9.1 to 0. We thus will observe pattern 2 results for all levels of confidence associated with t statistics ranging between Q/se_q and the t statistic defined by eqn 9.5. Finally, we will observe pattern 3 results for levels of confidence associated with t statistics that are greater than the t-statistic defined by eqn 9.5.

9.5.1. Special cases

Special cases occur at the boundary between patterns 1 and 2 (i.e., the level of confidence associated with the t statistic that equals Q/se_q) and the boundary between patterns 2 and 3 (i.e., the level of confidence associated with the t statistic defined in eqn 9.5). At the boundary between patterns 1 and 2, maximum willingnesses to pay fall into only two ranges: one range where we cannot be confident that the two strategies differ from one another and a second range where we can be confident that the strategy with either the larger or smaller point estimate for effect is good value, but not both. At the boundary between patterns 2 and 3, the middle range in pattern 2, which is where we can be confident that either the more effective strategy or the less effective strategy is good value, but not both, has shrunk to a single value of willingness to pay. For all other willingnesses to pay, we cannot be confident that the two strategies differ from one another.

Finally, the rooted term in the numerator and the denominator can both equal 0 at the same time. In this case, depending on our desired level of confidence, we can observe pattern 1 or pattern 3 findings, but we cannot observe any pattern 2 findings.

9.6. Undefined confidence intervals for cost-effectiveness ratios

If a dependably accurate 95% confidence interval covers truth 95% of the time and excludes truth 5% of the time, some might wonder how a method that can yield undefined confidence intervals, which cannot exclude truth, can be dependably accurate? Some might also wonder if there is additional information that we can provide to decision makers if the confidence interval for the cost-effectiveness ratio is undefined?

9.6.1. How can a method that yields undefined intervals be dependably accurate?

This question represents a misreading of the definition of dependably accurate 95% confidence intervals for cost-effectiveness ratios. A 95% confidence interval is dependably accurate if in repeated experiments, 95% have confidence intervals that cover truth (i.e., truth falls within the interval for 95% of the experiments) whereas 5% have confidence intervals that fail to cover truth (i.e., truth falls outside the interval for 5% of the experiments). The fact that in the current experiment the confidence interval is undefined indicates only that the current experiment is one of the 95% that covers truth. It provides no information about whether 95% of repeated experiments will cover truth.

Heitjan [5] has shown that even in the case where the Fieller's theorem method confidence interval for the cost-effectiveness ratio is undefined, a coverage experiment will demonstrate that the interval is dependably accurate. In such a coverage experiment, approximately 5% of the repeated experiments will have defined Fieller theorem method intervals that fail to cover truth; approximately 95% of the repeated experiments will have either a defined Fieller theorem method interval that covers truth or an undefined Fieller theorem method interval that by definition covers truth. Thus, to reiterate, the presence or absence of an undefined confidence interval says nothing about whether the Fieller theorem method produces dependably accurate confidence intervals.

9.6.2. Reporting when the confidence interval for the cost-effectiveness ratio is undefined

As we have indicated earlier, there is no more ambiguity in the confidence statements we derive from pattern 3 results – whether they are reported by use of confidence intervals for cost-effectiveness ratios, confidence intervals for NMB, or acceptability curves – than there is for the confidence statements we derive from patterns 1 and 2 results: there is no willingness to pay for which we can be 95% confident that the economic value of the two therapies differs. However, the fact that there are experiments like #3 in Chapter 8 for which a 95% confidence interval for the cost-effectiveness ratio cannot be defined is one of the reasons some may find confidence intervals for these ratios unsatisfactory. Thus, in cases where the confidence interval for the cost-effectiveness ratio is undefined, is there more information we can provide than simply reporting the lack of definition?

Additional information that might be useful would be to identify the confidence intervals whose limits equal policy-relevant maximum acceptable willingnesses to pay. For example, in experiment 3, the 25% confidence interval has an upper limit just under 30,000; the 46% confidence interval has an upper limit just under 50,000; and the 55% confidence interval has an upper limit just under 75,000. Thus, we can be 25% confident that therapy A is good value compared to therapy B if our maximum willingness to pay is 30,000; we can be 46% confident that it is good value if our maximum willingness to pay is 50,000; and we can be 55% confident if our maximum willingness to pay is 75,000. (There may be some decision makers for whom these levels of confidence are sufficient for selecting one therapy compared to another.) Alternatively, we may want to use eqn 9.5 to identify and report the largest definable confidence interval. The magnitude of this interval represents a kind of information statistic that defines the highest level of confidence about the difference in economic value between the two therapies that we can possibly derive from the experiment.

9.7. **Hypothesis testing**

Prior to the development of methods for assessing sampling uncertainty for the comparison of cost and effect, economists attempted to judge confidence by estimating the point estimate for the cost-effectiveness ratio and evaluating how these ratios varied in the face of sensitivity analysis. Development of methods for assessing uncertainty has changed the economic questions that can be asked about medical therapies. For example, rather than focusing on point estimate-based questions such as "Is the therapy cost-effective?", we can now focus on sampling uncertainty-based questions such as "how confident are we that the therapy is cost effective?" To address these latter questions, we can test hypotheses about expected cost-effectiveness ratios or NMB, for example that the incremental ratio of therapy X compared with therapy Y will be lower than W per QALY. These hypotheses may be tested by determining whether the confidence interval for the observed cost-effectiveness ratio excludes W; determining if the NMB calculated using a maximum willingness to pay of W is significantly greater than 0; or by calculating the probability that the observed ratio is acceptable.

9.7.1. **Sample size**

Because of its standard statistical properties, a number of authors have used the net benefit confidence limit equation to derive formulas for estimating sample size needed to test these hypotheses [8–11]. These formulas are derived from the statistical test of whether net benefit, calculated by use of W, is significantly different from 0. For example, if we assume that standard deviations of cost and effect differ between two treatment groups, we can use the following sample size formula for NMB:

$$n =$$

$$\frac{\left(t_{\alpha/2}+t_\beta\right)\left\{(sd_{c0}^2+sd_{c1}^2)+W^2(sd_{q0}^2+sd_{q1}^2)-2W\rho(sd_{c0}^2+sd_{c1}^2)^{0.5}(sd_{q0}^2+sd_{q1}^2)^{0.5}\right\}}{(WQ-C)^2}, \quad (9.6)$$

where n equals the sample size per group, sd_c0 and sd_c1 equal the standard deviation of cost for treatment groups 0 and 1, sd_q0 and sd_q0 equal the standard deviation of effect for these treatment groups, and t_β equals the t statistic for the planned type 2 error. Note that if we assume that the standard deviations for cost and effect are the same between the groups, we can represent their sums as $2sd_c^2$ and $2sd_q^2$.

9.7.2. Power

If you are working in a trial with a prespecified sample size, you may also be interested in the power you will have to rule out cost-effectiveness ratios that exceed the maximum willingness to pay. You can rearrange eqn 9.6 to obtain an estimate of the power of the study:

$$t_\beta =$$

$$\sqrt{\frac{n\times(WQ-C)^2}{\left\{(sd_{c0}^2+sd_{c1}^2)+W^2(sd_{q0}^2+sd_{q1}^2)-2W\rho(sd_{c0}^2+sd_{c1}^2)^{0.5}(sd_{q0}^2+sd_{q1}^2)^{0.5}\right\}}}-t_{\alpha/2} \quad (9.7)$$

Negative values of t_β represent power between 0 and 0.5; values greater than 0 represent power between 0.5 and 1.0 (e.g., −0.84 represents a power of approximately 0.2; 0 represents a power of 0.5; 0.84 represents a power of approximately 0.80).

9.7.3. Correlation

The correlation between the difference in cost and effect plays a potentially counterintuitive role in these calculations. All else equal, we need a relatively larger sample size to demonstrate that a therapy is good value if health care cost is lowest when the therapy is most effective and highest when it is least effective (referred to as win–win or negative correlation). An example of such a therapy might be a drug for asthma which reduces cost when it successfully avoids exacerbations and is associated with increased cost when it fails to avoid these exacerbations.

All else equal, we need a relatively smaller sample size to demonstrate that a therapy is good value if health care cost is highest when the therapy is more effective and lowest when it is least effective (referred to as win–lose or positive correlation). An example of such a therapy might be a treatment for stroke which leads to increased cost when it saves lives and leaves the survivors with costly rehabilitation and/or disability and leads to reduced cost when it fails to save lives.

Inspection of the sample size formula demonstrates this relationship. Correlation enters the term $(2W\rho(sd_{c0}^2 + sd_{c1}^2)^{0.5} (sd_{q0}^2 + sd_{q1}^2)^{0.5})$ in the numerator. When the correlation is positive, this term is subtracted from the numerator, which reduces the sample size necessary to demonstrate an economic difference between two therapies. When the correlation is negative, this term is added to the numerator, which increases the required sample size.

Figure 9.4 provides an extreme example of these relationships. The triangles represent the distribution of the difference in cost and effect for a hypothetical example of a therapy that has a win–lose correlation. The circles represent the distribution of the difference for a hypothetical example that is identical to the prior example in every way except for its having a win–win correlation. For identically sized trials, with identical estimates of the difference in cost and effect, and identical measures of variability, the therapy with the win–lose correlation is shown to be good value for lower maximum willingnesses to pay (dashed line confidence limits for the cost-effectiveness ratio ranging from 22,200 to 43,700), whereas we cannot be as confident about the value of the therapy with the win–win correlation (double dotted and dashed confidence limits ranging from 10,900 to 88,700).

9.8. **Decision rules and sampling uncertainty**

In the same way that the literature related to the assessment of sampling uncertainty has changed the economic questions we can ask, it has also changed how we interpret the results of economic evaluation.

In Chapter 7, we indicated that if we wish to select therapies but have not quantified sampling uncertainty, we need to calculate cost-effectiveness ratios or NMB when the differences in cost and effect are significant (guideline 1), but otherwise need not compare cost and effect. In other words, we need not

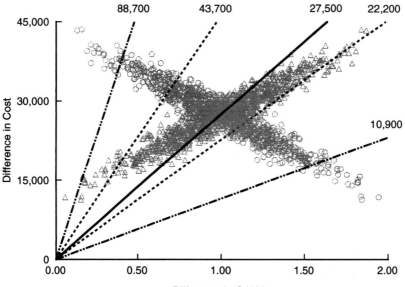

Fig. 9.4 Examples of win–win (negative) and win–lose (positive) correlation between the difference in cost and effect and its effect on statements of confidence. Open circles represent the distribution of the difference in cost and effect for the evaluation of a hypothetical therapy with win–win correlation; open triangles represent the distribution of the difference for the evaluation of a hypothetical therapy with win–lose correlation. For each comparison, differences in arithmetic mean cost and effect are identical (27,000 and 1 QALY) as are the measures of variability (standard errors for the difference in cost and effect, 5000 and 0.30, respectively) and sample size (250/group). The only difference between the experiments is in the correlation for the difference in cost and effect (triangles, 0.95; circles, –0.95). This difference in correlation leads to a widening of the resulting confidence interval for the cost-effectiveness ratio from a range of 22,200 to 43,700 (dashed confidence limits) for the therapy with win–lose correlation to a range of 10,900 to 88,700 (double dotted and dashed lines) for the therapy with win–win correlation.

compare cost and effect when one therapy's cost is significantly smaller and effect significantly larger than the other therapy's (guideline 2); when the two therapies' effect is not significantly different and one therapy has significantly lower cost (guideline 3, cost-minimization); when the two therapies' cost is not significantly different and one therapy has significantly larger effect (guideline 4, effect-maximization); or when the two therapies' cost and effect are not significantly different (guideline 5).

9.8.1. **Decision criteria that incorporate sampling uncertainty**

If we wish to take sampling uncertainty into account when making adoption decisions (e.g., to include confidence statements in these decisions), we need to modify a number of these guidelines. For example, a finding of no significant difference in effect but a significant reduction in cost (guideline 3) need not guarantee that we can be 95% confident that the significantly less expensive therapy is good value. Suppose you conducted an experiment with 250 participants per treatment group and found a significant difference in cost of −500 (SE, 200; $p = 0.01$), a nonsignificant difference in effect of 0.01 QALYs (SE, 0.03; $p = 0.74$; 95% CI, −0.05 to 0.07), and a correlation of the difference in cost and effect of 0. The resulting lower confidence limit for this pattern 2 experiment would be 9400; the resulting upper confidence limit would be -3000. The negative upper limit indicates that the significantly less expensive therapy might dominate the alternative (i.e., it might save money and improve effect). However, the positive lower limit indicates that we cannot rule out that the alternative may cost more and do more than the significantly less expensive therapy, and when it does, we cannot rule out with 95% confidence that it is producing the additional QALYs for as little as 9400 per QALY. Thus, guideline 3, which recommends the adoption of cost-minimization analysis without the comparison of cost and effect, can no longer be supported once we introduce sampling uncertainty.

Similar reasoning undermines guideline 4, which recommends effect-maximization when there is no significant difference in cost but a significant improvement in effect. Suppose you conducted an experiment with 250 participants per treatment group and found a nonsignificant difference in cost of 800 (SE, 2500; $p = 0.75$; 95% CI, −4100 to 5700), a significant difference in effect of 0.05 QALYs (SE, 0.02; $p = 0.01$), and a correlation of the difference in cost and effect of 0.25. The resulting confidence interval for this pattern 1 experiment would range from −165,600 in the lower right quadrant to 148,400 in the upper right quadrant. The negative lower limit indicates that the significantly more effective therapy might dominate the alternative (i.e., it might save money and improve effect). However, the upper limit indicates that we cannot rule out with 95% confidence that the significantly more effective therapy costs as much as 148,400 per QALY gained.

Results like those for the last two experiments arise in part because the initial guidelines conflated the ideas of "absence of evidence of a difference" and "evidence of absence of a difference." These experiments do not allow us to be confident that the effect (first experiment) or cost (second experiment) is actually the same between the two therapies. They are representative of experiments that provide an absence of evidence. Thus, the resulting confidence intervals for the cost-effectiveness ratio are wide and undermine the use of cost-minimization or effect-maximization. Had we instead been more confident that these therapies do not differ in their effect or in their cost – for example, from evidence from clinical equivalence trials that attempt to rule out excessively large differences between therapies, and thus provide evidence of absence of difference – our confidence intervals would have been substantially narrower than the ones we observed, and we may have had sufficient evidence to be confident about value for the cost.

Introduction of sampling uncertainty probably has its most counterintuitive effect on guideline 5, which recommends against evaluation of cost effectiveness when there is no significant difference in cost or effect. Experiments 1 and 2 from Chapter 8 illustrate the difference well. Recall that in experiment 1, therapy A costs significantly more and was significantly more effective than therapy B and had a point estimate for the cost-effectiveness ratio of 100,000. In experiment 2, there was no significant difference in cost or effect between therapies A and B, but the point estimate for the cost-effectiveness ratio was 875.

For experiment 1, if we followed guideline 1 from Chapter 7, for willingnesses to pay in the range of 30,000 – 75,000, we would conclude that therapy A is not good value, because the point estimate for the cost-effectiveness ratio exceeds our maximum willingness to pay. If we assessed sampling uncertainty, we would conclude that we cannot be 95% confident that therapies A and B differ in their value, because our willingness to pay falls within the resulting 95% confidence interval. For experiment 2, if we followed guideline 5 from Chapter 7, we would stop our evaluation after we found no significant difference in cost or effect. However, as we indicated in Chapter 8, when we consider sampling uncertainty for experiment 2, if our maximum willingness to pay falls in the range between 28,200 and 245,200, we can be 95% confident that therapy A is good value compared to therapy B, even though neither its cost nor effect were significantly different than therapy B's.

What has the introduction of sampling uncertainty changed so dramatically that not only is it wrong for us to omit comparison of cost and effect when there are no significant differences between the therapies, but these may be the experiments where we can recommend one therapy compared to another? The answer is that the introduction of sampling uncertainty for the comparison of cost and effect allows us to take advantage of the power to detect a difference in the joint cost–effect outcome. In some cases, the power to detect a difference in this joint outcome exceeds the power to detect differences in either cost or effect alone.

This issue of joint versus independent significance is widely acknowledged in other areas of medical research. For example, it is common to find clinical trials in which a therapy's clinical effect on nonfatal events is nonsignificant as is its clinical effect on fatal events, yet its effect on nonfatal and fatal events jointly is significant. In our case, cost and effect are like nonfatal and fatal events, but they are combined either by use of a cost-effectiveness ratio or by a summation of the differences by use of NMB.

More guideline 5 examples

Figures 9.5A–C provide examples of three pattern 2 experiments that have no significant difference in either cost or effect, and thus would be subject to the guideline 5 recommendation from chapter 7 that we need not compare cost and effect. Two of these experiments represent cases where – given maximum willingnesses to pay between 30,000 and 75,000 – we cannot be 95% confident that the therapies differ in their economic value, and for these experiments guideline 5 might be considered to have been appropriate. In one, we can be 95% confident that the therapy with the larger point estimate for effect is good value, in which case the guideline is inappropriate.

The first experiment (Fig. 9.5A) represents the case where the entire upper right quadrant of the cost-effectiveness plane is included in the confidence interval. Because the upper right quadrant contains all positive values of willingness to pay, and because the entire quadrant is included within the confidence interval, this experiment does not allow us to be 95% confident that the therapies differ in their economic value. In addition, because the limits fall in the lower right and upper left quadrants, we cannot rule out with 95% confidence that therapy A dominates therapy B or that therapy B dominates therapy A.

In the second experiment (Fig. 9.5B), the 95% confidence interval for the cost-effectiveness ratio ranges from -∞ to 5000 and from 19,800 to ∞. It excludes ratios between 5000 and 19,800. Thus, if our willingness to pay falls in the latter range, we can be 95% confident that the therapy with the larger point estimate for effectiveness is good value. If our maximum willingness to pay is larger than 19,800 or smaller than 5000, we cannot be 95% confident that the economic value of the therapies differs. This lack of confidence is because the latter two ranges of willingness to pay are included in the confidence interval.

Finally, the third experiment (Fig. 9.5C) represents the case where the 95% confidence interval for the cost-effectiveness ratio ranges from —∞ to 7200 and from 615,000 to ∞. Ratios between 7200 and 615,000 on the other hand are excluded from the interval. In this case, if our maximum willingness to pay

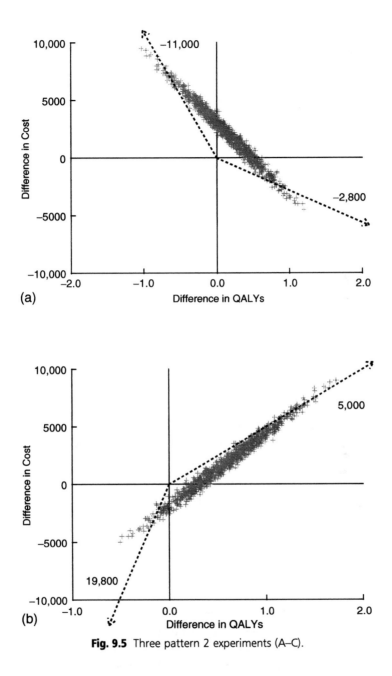

Fig. 9.5 Three pattern 2 experiments (A–C).

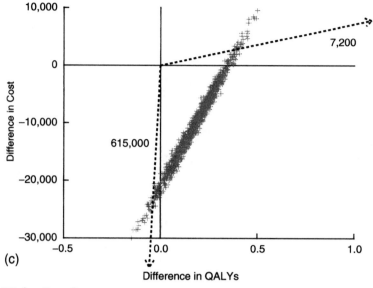

Fig. 9.5 (continued)

ranges between 7200 and 615,000 we can be 95% confident that the therapy
with the larger point estimate of effectiveness is good value. Thus, we observe
an experiment in which there is no significant difference in cost and effect, yet
guideline 5 provides bad advice.

What then are the revised guidelines for therapy selection in the light of
sampling uncertainty?

(1) If one therapy's cost is significantly smaller and its effect significantly
    larger than another's, adopt this dominant therapy. We need not calculate
    a cost-effectiveness ratio or its confidence interval, because they will all be
    negative and will restate the finding of dominance.

(2) For all other combinations of significance or lack thereof for cost and
    effect, calculate a cost-effectiveness ratio or NMB and their confidence
    intervals.

Sampling uncertainty also affects the algorithm for choosing among more
than two therapies that we described in Table 7.2 in Chapter 7. Recall that in
step 2 of this algorithm, we eliminated therapies that were strongly dominated
by at least one other therapy; in step 4 we eliminated therapies that were
weakly dominated. Although little has been written about this issue, once we
account for sampling uncertainty, therapies should only be eliminated if they
are significantly strongly or weakly dominated.

9.9. **Symmetry of the acceptability criterion in the upper right and lower left quadrants**

We drew the acceptability criteria in Fig. 9.2 as lines through the origin with slopes that define willingnesses to pay (and to accept). When drawn as lines through the origin, they presume that we are willing to pay the same amount to gain health as we are willing to save to give up health. In other words, they presume that if we would not spend more than $50,000 per QALY gained for a more costly and more effective new therapy in the upper right quadrant, then we would be willing to forego QALYs if we saved 50,000 or more per QALY for a less costly and less effective alternative in the lower left quadrant. Some have suggested that preferences for gains and losses of health are asymmetric [12,13]. Confidence interval for cost-effectiveness ratios are probably least affected by such asymmetries. They can be incorporated into the acceptability criterion by allowing the slopes of the rays representing acceptable ratios in the upper right and lower left quadrants to differ. Note that this issue complicates the interpretation of these curves, and complicates both the construction of 95% CI for, and the interpretation of, NMB.

9.10. **Negative cost-effectiveness ratios**

When one therapy costs less and is more effective than another, the point estimate for its cost-effectiveness ratio will be negative. Similarly, when a sufficient fraction of the distribution of the difference in cost and effect falls in the lower right or upper left quadrants, one or both confidence limits can fall in these quadrants and be negative. Given that negative ratios do not report trade-offs between cost and effect in the same way that positive ratios do [14], should we report the magnitude of negative ratios, or should we simply report that they are negative and provide the appropriate interpretation that they provide evidence of dominance or of being dominated?

One problem with reporting negative point estimates for cost-effectiveness ratios is that their relative magnitude says nothing about whether a therapy with a larger negative ratio is better or worse than a therapy with a smaller negative ratio. For example, points on a ray from the origin in the lower right quadrant, which defines a single ratio, dominate one another as we move further from the origin. For example, in Fig. 9.6, A and B have the same negative cost-effectiveness ratio, but A dominates B because A is both less expensive and more effective. In addition, pairs of points in these quadrants can be defined such that in one pair, the point with the less negative ratio dominates the point with the more negative ratio, whereas in the other pair, the opposite is true. For example, A, with the less negative ratio, dominates C, with the

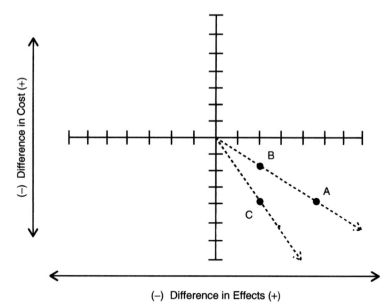

Fig. 9.6 Examples of negative ratios whose relative magnitudes say nothing about whether a therapy with a larger negative ratio is better or worse than a therapy with a smaller ratio.

more negative ratio, but C, with the more negative ratio, dominates B, with the less negative ratio. Thus, the magnitude of negative point estimates of ratios in the same quadrant does not provide information about the relative preferability of these different therapies.

There is somewhat more information in negative confidence intervals for cost-effectiveness ratios, but even so, it is unlikely that anything is gained by reporting the magnitudes of the negative confidence intervals. For example, consider two experiments, one with a confidence interval that ranges from a lower limit of −11,000 to −2800, the other with a confidence interval that ranges from a lower limit of −2800 to −11,000 (as in Fig. 9.5A). Because the lower limit in the first experiment is smaller than the upper limit, we can conclude that we are observing a pattern 1 result. Given that the only willingnesses to pay that fall within this interval are between −11,000 and −2800, we can be 95% confident that the therapy with the larger point estimate for effectiveness significantly dominates the alternative for all positive willingnesses to pay. Once we report the fact that the confidence interval confirms a finding of dominance, however, it is not clear that anything is gained by reporting the magnitudes of the negative limits.

Because the lower limit in the second experiment is larger than the upper limit, we can conclude that we are observing a pattern 2 finding. The interval for this experiment includes all willingnesses to pay except those between −2800 and −11,000. Because all positive willingnesses to pay fall within this interval, we cannot be 95% confident that the economic value of the two therapies differs. But as with the first experiment above, once we report the fact that the confidence intervals indicate we cannot be confident that the two therapies differ, it is not clear that anything is gained by reporting the magnitudes of the negative limits.

9.11. **Recommendations**

When reporting sampling uncertainty related to the comparison of cost and effect, consider showing the distribution of the difference in cost and effect on the cost-effectiveness plane either by plotting confidence ellipses from the joint normal distribution or by plotting bootstrap replicates (see many of the figures in Chapters 8 and 9). One reason to do so is that this distribution telegraphs much of the economic information from the experiment, without the potentially counterintuitive results from cost-effectiveness ratios, NMB, or acceptability curves.

When you are observing a pattern 1 result, interpretation is straightforward, no matter which method you choose to quantify sampling uncertainty. If you are observing a pattern 2 or 3 result, on the other hand, be prepared to provide detailed information to help your reader understand your results. For example, consider reporting ranges of cost-effectiveness where your audience can and cannot be confident about adopting a therapy rather than simply reporting (1) a confidence interval for the cost-effectiveness ratio whose lower limit is greater than its upper limit, (2) confidence intervals for NMB that always include 0, and (3) acceptability curves that never are below 0.025 or exceed 0.975.

Finally, to again reiterate one of the conclusions from Chapter 8, the confidence statements you derive from an experiment will be the same whether you quantify sampling uncertainty by use of confidence intervals for cost-effectiveness analysis, NMB, or acceptability curves. More research is needed to determine if one or the other of these methods is more easily understood or better accepted by the audience to whom you wish to communicate your results.

References

1. **Fieller EC.** Some problems in interval estimation with discussion. *J Roy Stat Soc Series B.* 1954; 16: 175–88.
2. **Chaudhary MA, Stearns SC.** Estimating confidence intervals for cost-effectiveness ratios: an example from a randomized trial. *Stat Med.* 1996; 15: 1447–58.

3. **Willan AR, O'Brien BJ.** Confidence intervals for cost-effectiveness ratios: an application of Fieller's theorem. *Health Econ.* 1996; 5: 297–305.

4. **Polsky DP, Glick HA, Willke R, Schulman K.** Confidence intervals for cost-effectiveness ratios: a comparison of four methods. *Health Econ.* 1997; 6: 243–52.

5. **Heitjan DF.** Fieller's method and net health benefits. *Health Econ.* 2000; 9: 327–35.

6. **Efron B, Tibshirani RJ.** An Introduction to the Bootstrap. New York: Chapman and Hall, 1993.

7. **Briggs AH, Wonderling DE, Moony CZ.** Pulling cost-effectiveness analysis up by its bootstraps: a non-parametric approach to confidence interval estimation. *Health Econ.* 1997; 6: 327–40.

8. **Willan AR, O'Brien BJ.** Sample size and power issues in estimating incremental cost-effectiveness ratios from clinical trials data. *Health Econ.* 1999; 8: 203–11.

9. **Laska EM, Meisner M, Seigel C.** Power and sample size in cost-effectiveness analysis. *Med Decis Making* 1999; 19: 339–43.

10. **Briggs AH, Gray AM.** Power and sample size calculations for stochastic cost-effectiveness analysis. *Med Decis Making* 1998; 18: S81–92.

11. **Al MJ, van Hout BA, Rutten FFH.** Sample size calculations in economic evaluations. *Health Econ.* 1998; 7: 327–35.

12. **Viscusi WK, Magat WA, Scharff R.** Asymmetric assessments in valuing pharmaceutical risks. *Med Care* 1996; 34: DS34–47.

13. **O'Brien BJ, Gertsen K, Willan AR, Faulkner LA.** Is there a kink in consumers' threshold value for cost-effectiveness in health care? *Health Econ.* 2002; 11: 175–80.

14. **Stinnett AA, Mullahy J.** The negative side of cost-effectiveness analysis. *JAMA.* 1997; 277: 1931–32.

Chapter 10

Transferability of the results from trials

In Chapters 7–9, we have discussed the comparison of cost and effect and sampling uncertainty surrounding this comparison. In this chapter, we discuss a second form of uncertainty: to whom does the resulting trial-wide – or pooled – cost-effectiveness ratio apply. This issue has been referred to in the literature as transferability [1] or generalizability [2]. In what follows, we identify problems confronting the interpretation of economic results from multinational trials; review several inadequate solutions to the problem; summarize current evidence about which is more important for transferability, medical service use or price weights; review three analytic approaches for the evaluation of transferability; and identify issues that potentially pose problems for all three methods.

10.1. The problem

Multicenter and multinational trials are the norm for the evaluation of new medical therapies. They speed the development process, broaden the representativeness of the patients who receive the therapy, and familiarize clinical decision makers with the therapy prior to its approval by regulatory agencies. At the same time, they can increase the heterogeneity of patients, disease presentation and severity, medical service use, price weights, and the like that are observed in the trial. While this increased heterogeneity can occur for both multicenter trials that are conducted within a single country and for multinational trials, in this chapter we focus on the latter set of issues. Many of the lessons that we learn for multinational trials will apply equally to multicenter trials.

The presence of between-country heterogeneity in trials has led to a growing concern that the pooled or average economic results from multinational trials may not be reflective of the results that would be observed in individual countries that participated in the trial. Common sources for concern about the representativeness of data from multinational trials include transnational differences in morbidity/mortality patterns; practice patterns (i.e., medical service use); and absolute and relative prices for medical service use (i.e., price weights).

Thus, decision makers may find it difficult to draw conclusions about the value for the cost of the therapies that are evaluated in multinational trials.

At the same time, as O'Brien [1] has noted, it is impossible to replicate trials in all settings where therapy choices are made. Thus, there is a need to use the data we collect in multinational trials to provide decision makers in individual countries with information they can use in making adoption decisions.

Concerns about transferability may arise due to variations in underlying morbidity/mortality patterns in different countries. For example, the cost-effectiveness of cholesterol-lowering agents may vary if the underlying risk for coronary heart disease differs. Potential sources of variation include naturally occurring differences, differences in disease identification and treatment, and variation in severities of disease of enrolled participants between countries, which sometimes is referred to as cream-skimming or reverse cream-skimming.

Concerns about transferability may also arise due to variations in practice patterns in different countries. Effectiveness of a therapy may be related to the other care received by participants. Thus, if the therapy is complementary with other supportive care, i.e., if it is more effective when combined with other supportive care, it will be more cost-effective in countries that provide more supportive care and less cost-effective in countries that provide less of it. Alternatively, if the therapy substitutes for other supportive care, i.e., if it is more effective when this other care is absent, the reverse will be true.

Of note, one sometimes hears the converse argument made about economic data from multinational trials. The concern expressed is that the protocol may be so prescriptive about the care provided to participants that the trial does not allow us to observe differences between countries. While such protocol-induced care may diminish observed between-country differences, in our experience the protocol usually does not eliminate all differences in country-specific medical service use. For example, when we assessed differences in this use and clinical outcomes observed in a stroke trial conducted in Canada and the U.S., we found significant differences between the average length of hospital stay in Canada and the U.S.; the proportion of the stay that was spent in routine care and intensive care units; the use of nursing homes and rehabilitation centers; and the cost of the episode of care. On the other hand, we found no statistically significant differences in outcomes between participants treated in the two countries [3].

Finally, concerns about transferability also arise because of absolute and relative differences in price weights between countries. For example, when addressing transferability of data from other countries, Australian, Canadian, and British guidelines for cost-effectiveness [4–6] all request that local price weights be used in evaluations submitted to the government, and at least one has a preferred schedule for such submissions. However, there is little evidence about the impact of simply valuing trial-wide medical service use by use of country-specific price weights (referred to by Reed *et al.* [7] as fully pooled, one-country costing). For example, when Willke *et al.* [2] evaluated this impact in a European stroke trial, they found that when one estimated five different cost-effectiveness ratios by valuing trial-wide medical services by use of five sets of country-specific price weights (the second of the four columns in Table 10.1), there was little to no variability in the point estimates for the resulting cost-effectiveness ratio. For example, when country 1's price weights were used to value trial-wide medical service use, the cost-effectiveness ratio equaled 46,800. When country 5's price weights were used to value this same medical service use the ratio equaled 69,100.

This last solution – using trial-wide clinical results, trial-wide medical service use, and price weights from a single country – is one of the commonly proposed, potentially inadequate solutions to the problem of transferability (e.g., to tailor the results to the U.K., simply use U.K. price weights, and conduct the analysis as if all participants were treated in the U.K.). A second potentially inadequate solution is to use trial-wide clinical results, and country-specific medical service use and price weights (referred to by Reed *et al.* [7] as partially split, one-country costing). Both approaches have the failing that they ignore the fact that clinical and economic outcomes may influence one another. That is, differences in cost may affect practice patterns, which in turn may affect outcome; differences in practice pattern may affect outcome, which in turn may affect cost.

Table 10.1 Impact of price weight and service use variation on country-specific cost-effectiveness ratios

| Country | Trial-wide effect | | Country- specific cost and effect |
	Price weights*	Country-specific cost†	
1	46,800	5900	11,500
2	53,900	90,500	244,100
3	57,600	91,900	60,400
4	65,800	**	**
5	69,100	93,300	181,300
Overall	45,900	45,900	45,900

*Trial-wide resource use × country-specific price weights.
†Country-specific resource use × country-specific price weights.
**New therapy dominates.

10.2. **Relative impact of medical service use and price weights**

What do we know about whether medical service use or price weights have a greater impact on transferability of results of trials? Returning to the data in Table 10.1, Willke *et al.* [2] evaluated the relative impact of medical service use and price weights by calculating cost-effectiveness ratios for five countries by use of (a) trial-wide clinical outcome and medical service use and country-specific price weights (column 2), (b) trial-wide clinical outcome and country-specific medical service use and price weights (column 3), and (c) country-specific clinical outcome, medical service use, and price weights (column 4). As we noted above, when the authors allowed price weights alone to vary between countries, there was little variation in the resulting cost-effectiveness ratios. When they allowed medical service use and price weights to vary, there was substantially more variation (ranging from dominance in one country to ratios of 90,000+ per death averted in three countries). Finally, when they allowed clinical outcome, medical service use, and price weights to vary they observed the greatest variability (ranging from dominance to 244,100 per death averted). Thus, in this one study, price weights had little impact on the observed cost-effectiveness ratio, whereas medical service use and, particularly, clinical outcome had a substantial effect on the ratio.

In a second study, Barbieri *et al.* [8] attempted to identify the major causes of variation in study results between countries. The authors conducted a literature search by use of OHE-HEED [9] and NHS EED [10] to identify economic evaluations of pharmaceuticals that were conducted in two or more European countries and were published between January 1988 and December 2001. As with the Willke study, the authors classified studies by whether price weights, price weights and medical service use, or price weights, medical service use, and clinical effect were allowed to vary in the analysis. They also classified the studies by the level of variability of the results between countries. They referred to studies as having "low variability" if they judged that the observed differences in incremental cost-effectiveness ratios were unlikely to change adoption decisions in different countries; they referred to studies as having "high variability" if they judged that the observed differences in incremental cost-effectiveness ratios were likely to change the adoption decision.

Barbieri *et al.* [8] identified 44 studies that had sufficient country-specific data for inclusion in their analysis. As indicated in Fig. 10.1, they found that 84% (16/19) of studies that allowed only price weights to vary had low variability, i.e., they would likely lead to similar recommendations in all countries; 62.5% (5/8) of studies that allowed price weights and medical service use to

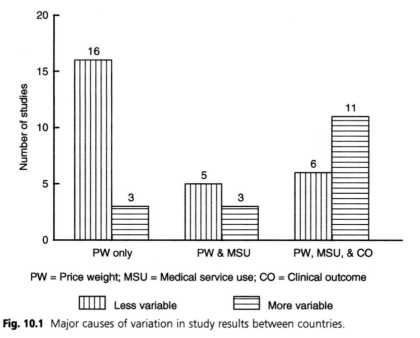

Fig. 10.1 Major causes of variation in study results between countries.

vary would likely lead to similar recommendations in all countries; whereas only 35% (6/17) of studies that allowed price weights, medical service use, and clinical effect to vary would likely lead to similar recommendations. They concluded that the amount of variation in study results that was observed across countries depended upon the amount of variation that was allowed by the studies' authors. In particular, they identified as a key factor whether the authors of trial-based studies allowed medical service use to vary across countries.

While both of these studies lend support to the idea that when we transfer results to countries with similar levels of economic development medical service use matters more than price weights, they both also share a common weakness that may diminish the strength of this conclusion. The results based on trial-wide medical service use and country-specific price weights use the entire sample to estimate each country-specific cost-effectiveness ratio. The results based on country-specific medical service use and price weights use the – potentially – much smaller country-specific sample sizes to estimate each country-specific ratio. The weakness is that whenever we subdivide a larger group into smaller groups, we should expect to observe increases in the variability in the point estimates, even if medical service use were identical in all countries.

For example, when countries' medical service use has the same mean and variance and the countries differ in their price weights alone, the expected difference in variability associated with use of country-specific rather than trial-wide medical service use equals $(N_T^{0.5}/N_i^{0.5})$, where N_T represents the total number of participants in the trial and N_i represents the number of participants in country i. For example, if there are 100 participants in each of two countries, the standard errors for the estimates derived from country-specific medical service use and price weights would be 41% $((N_T^{0.5}/N_i^{0.5}))$ = (14.142136/10) greater than those derived from trial-wide medical service use and country-specific price weights. If, on the other hand, the means and variances for medical service use differ between countries, the variability can increase even further.

What then can we conclude from the studies of Willke *et al.* and Barbieri *et al.*? One observation that does not seem in doubt is that if we are working in countries with similar economic conditions (e.g., Western Europe), multiplication of trial-wide medical service use times a country's price weights tends to shrink estimates for all countries towards a common result. Whether or not medical service use matters more than price weights is a matter of conjecture, although the current evidence does not rule out this possibility. Better evaluations, which overcome the problem of the different sample sizes, are needed before we can draw reliable conclusions.

10.3. **Analytic approaches to transferability**

If multiplication of trial-wide service use times country-specific price weights is a flawed method for assessing transferability, how should we make such assessments? In this section, we describe three proposed statistical methods that use patient-level data to address transferability: fixed effects models [2], tests of homogeneity [11], and multilevel models with random effects empirical Bayesian shrinkage estimators [12–14]. All three share the common approach of using country-specific data for the estimates, although the random effects models also borrow information from the pooled study result to overcome the problem of the expected increase in variability that one observes when subsetting the data by country. While other methods for addressing transferability exist, including use of decision analysis [15] or combinations of decision analysis and patient-level data [16,17], these are not the focus of our discussion.

10.3.1. **Fixed effects models**

Willke *et al.* [2] proposed use of a fixed effects model to separate the study therapy's effect on cost (and effect) into two parts. The first is its direct effect on cost by changing medical service use independent of the clinical outcome; the second is its indirect effect on cost by changing the clinical outcome.

Underlying this separation is the assumption that cost for an individual participant may be affected by the study therapy the participant receives, a series of other variables such as age, gender, and disease severity that modify treatment and outcome, and the eventual health outcome. The model incorporates a number of therapy-by-country and country-by-outcome interaction terms that allow therapy to affect the cost independent of outcome (i.e., for two identical individuals who experience the same outcome, one with the study therapy and the other with usual care, the study therapy may cause the cost of care to differ). They also allow outcome to affect the cost of care, independent of study therapy (i.e., two identical individuals may experience different outcomes due to the study treatment and thus incur different cost). It further differentiates these independent effects by country.

This method proceeds by use of two sets of predictions. In the first, we estimate the effect of study therapy on outcome by use of linear prediction, logit, or probit models. For example, Willke et al. [2] estimated the probability of death via a probit. For this prediction, therapy-by-country interaction terms are used to allow the effect of the study therapy to vary between countries. In the second set of predictions, we estimate the effect of study therapy on cost, controlling for both outcome and the study therapy's effect on outcome. As with the first set of predictions, we not only include therapy-by-country interactions, but also include country-by-outcome interactions. The net result of the prediction combines the therapy's effect on cost through its effect – in the Willke example, on death – and its effect on cost independent of death.

The advantage of this approach is that it uses patient-level data and standard empirical procedures to identity country-specific differences in both cost and effect. It also enables sensitivity analyses, particularly with respect to country-specific treatment outcomes. On the other hand, this method's use of fixed effects models does not allow for the potentially hierarchical nature of the cost (and effect) data in multinational clinical trials [12]. Failure to account for the clustering that can exist within each country will result in overestimates of the precision and biased standard errors.

10.3.2. **Tests of homogeneity**

A second approach to the evaluation of transferability is to assess the homogeneity of the cost-effectiveness results from the different countries [11]. This evaluation is conducted by testing a series of treatment-by-country interaction terms to determine if there is evidence of between-country differences in the economic value of the therapy. If there is no evidence of heterogeneity (i.e., a nonsignificant p value for the test of homogeneity), and if we believe the test is powerful enough to rule out economically meaningful differences in cost, then we cannot reject that the pooled economic result from the trial applies to all of the countries that participated in the trial. If, on the other hand, there is evidence of heterogeneity, then the method indicates we should not use the pooled estimate to represent the result for the individual countries. When such a finding occurs, the method is less clear about the estimate we should use for an individual country.

Homogeneity of clinical effect

Clinical investigators have long recognized the need to evaluate the homogeneity of clinical effect observed in multinational trials. Commonly reported tests evaluate whether the treatment effect differs by gender, age, or disease severity. A number of methods are available for assessing whether the treatment effect is homogeneous. For example, one can use F or chi-square tests to determine whether a set of treatment-by-subgroup interaction terms are statistically significant.

Gail and Simon [18] have proposed decomposing these tests of interaction to determine whether the treatment effect is inconsistent in both direction and magnitude or whether it is consistent in direction but not in magnitude. They defined a qualitative or crossover interaction as one where the treatment effect is positive for the participants in some countries, and negative in other countries (i.e., inconsistent in both direction and magnitude). They defined a non-crossover interaction as one where there is variation in the magnitude of the effect, but not in its direction. For this type of interaction, the treatment effect may be positive in all countries, but it is more positive in some countries than in others. This latter type of interaction has also been termed a quantitative interaction [19].

We can test for qualitative interaction by using estimates of the treatment effect and its variance for each of the subgroups being evaluated (see Box 10.1 for a more detailed description). Our null hypothesis is that these effects are either all greater than 0 or all less than 0, and the statistical test is based on a likelihood ratio, with critical values of the test shown in Table B 10.1 in Box 10.1. The power of the test has been described by Pan and Wolfe [20].

We can test for quantitative interaction by use of the sum of squared errors of the subgroup-specific treatment effects and the variance of these effects. The test statistic is compared to critical values of the chi-square distribution with one less degree of freedom than there are subgroups being evaluated.

Independent test of the homogeneity of cost and effect

One approach to the evaluation of transferability might be to test the homogeneity of a therapy's independent impact on cost and effect. Under this

Box 10.1 Testing for qualitative and quantitative interactions

Defnitions

Treatment effect: D_i, where i = countries 1 to K, are estimates of the actual treatment effect (δ_i).

Variance of the treatment effect: S_i^2, where i = countries 1 to K.

Statistical test for qualitative interactions

Null hypothesis: All δ_i are either greater than 0 or they are all less than 0. Compute the following quantities:

$$Q^- = \sum_{i=1}^{k} (D_i^2 / S_i^2) \; \forall D_i > 0$$

$$Q^+ = \sum_{i=1}^{k} (D_i^2 / S_i^2) \; \forall D_i > 0$$

The likelihood ratio is expressed by:

$$Q = \min(Q^+, Q^-) > c$$

Critical values for c are given in Table B10.1.1 [18].

Table B10.1.1 Critical values (c) for the likelihood ratio test: min (Q^+, Q^-) > c

Number of groups	*p* Values			
	0.10	0.05	0.025	0.001
2	1.64	2.71	3.84	9.55
3	2.95	4.23	5.54	11.76
4	4.01	5.43	6.86	13.47
5	4.96	6.50	8.02	14.95
6	5.84	7.48	9.09	16.32
7	6.67	8.41	10.09	17.85
8	7.48	9.29	11.05	18.78
9	8.26	10.15	11.98	19.93
10	9.02	10.99	12.87	21.03
12	10.50	12.60	14.57	23.13

Box 10.1 Testing for qualitative and quantitative interactions *(continued)*

Table B10.1.1 Critical values (c) for the likelihood ratio test: min $(Q^+, Q^-) > c$

Number of groups	p Values			
	0.10	0.05	0.025	0.001
14	11.93	14.15	16.25	25.17
16	13.33	15.66	17.85	27.10
18	14.70	17.13	19.41	28.96
20	16.04	18.57	20.94	30.79
25	19.34	22.09	24.65	35.15
30	22.55	25.50	28.23	39.33

Source: From Gail M, Simon R. Testing for qualitative interactions between treatment effects and patient subsets. *Biometrics*. 1985; 41: 361–72. Permission sought from the International Biometrics Society.

Statistical test for quantitative interactions

Null hypothesis: All δ_i are equal.
Compute the following quantity:

$$H = \sum_{i-1}^{k}(D_i - \overline{D})^2 / S_i^2,$$

where

$$\overline{D} = \left[\sum_{i-1}^{k} D_i / S_i^2\right] / \left[\sum_{i-1}^{k} 1/S_i^2\right]$$

Computed values of H are compared to critical values of the x^2 distribution with K–1 degrees of freedom. Large values of H indicate heterogeneity.

approach, if there is no evidence that the therapy's impact on these outcomes differs by country, we might conclude that there is no evidence that its value for the cost is heterogeneous. Unfortunately, a finding of homogeneity of a therapy's independent impacts on cost and effect need not guarantee the homogeneity of the therapy's resulting cost-effectiveness ratio or net monetary benefit (NMB). Statistical tests of the clinical endpoints of trials often are based on relative measures such as odds ratios, hazard ratios, or relative risks. Cost-effectiveness ratios, on the other hand, are computed as the ratio of absolute differences in cost and outcome. See Box 10.2 for an example of

Box 10.2 Homogeneous odds ratios, heterogeneous cost-effectiveness ratios

Suppose you had data from two trials (see Table B10.2.1). Each trial was conducted in two countries, and in each trial the probability of the death among those receiving therapy A ($p\text{Death}_A$) is 20% in country 1 and 10% ($p < 0.05$) in country 2. In the first trial, the odds ratio for death among those receiving therapy B is 0.5 in both countries, and the homogeneity test indicates there is no evidence that these odds ratios differ. In the second trial, the odds ratio for death for those receiving therapy B is 0.72 in country 1 and 0.5 in country 2. The test of homogeneity indicates the two odds ratios differ ($p < 0.05$).

As shown in the table, trial 1, with the common odds ratio, is the trial in which there are absolute differences in avoided deaths between countries 1 and 2 (9.9% versus 4.7%) (i.e., if the denominator had been deaths averted, there would be more deaths averted in country 1 than in country 2). Trial 2, with the heterogeneous odds ratio, is the trial in which there is no absolute difference in country-specific avoided deaths (4.7% in both countries 1 and 2). Thus, homogeneity of relative treatment effect does not guarantee homogeneity of absolute treatment effect, and it is measures of absolute treatment effect that make up the numerator and denominator of the cost-effectiveness ratio.

Table B10.2.1 Risks for death, odds ratios, and deaths averted when country-specific mortality rates vary and their are common or heterogeneous country-specific odds ratios for death

Country	$p\text{Death}_A$	Odds ratio	$p\text{Death}_B$[†]	Avoided death $(p\text{Death}_A - p\text{Death}_B)$
Trial 1				
1	0.2	0.5	0.111	0.099
2	0.1	0.5	0.053	0.047
p value	< 0.05	~1.0	–	–
Trial 2				
1	0.2	0.72	0.153	0.047
2	0.1	0.5	0.053	0.047
p value	< 0.05	< 0.05	–	–

[†]$p\text{Death}_B = (p\text{Death}_A \times OR)/[(p\text{Death}_A \times OR) + (1 - p\text{Death}_A)]$

homogeneous odds ratios that occur in conjunction with variation in the placebo event rate which lead to differences in cost-effectiveness ratios.

Homogeneity of NMB

Instead of separately evaluating the homogeneity of a therapy's cost and effect, Cook et al. [11] proposed use of the Gail and Simon tests to determine whether there is evidence of heterogeneity in cost-effectiveness or NMB between the different countries that participated in the trial. The test for qualitative interaction determines whether the therapy has an NMB greater than 0 in some countries and less than 0 in others. The test for quantitative interaction determines whether the therapy has positive (negative) NMB in all countries, but differs in the magnitude of this positive (negative) NMB between the different countries.

In conducting these tests, Cook et al. [11] indicated that the estimate of treatment effect (e.g., NMB) and variance for each country should be derived separately and independently. If covariates are available, then they can be the estimated parameters from a regression model (e.g., GLM, linear, logistic, Poisson), or from a survival model (e.g., Cox Proportional Hazards Model). Note that while Cook et al. [11] suggested that homogeneity tests can be conducted either for cost-effectiveness ratios or NMBs, the fact that standard errors for the ratios need not always be defined suggests that these tests be limited to the evaluation of the homogeneity of NMB.

Heart failure example

Data for this example of an evaluation of a treatment-by-country interaction for NMB are drawn from a randomized, double-blinded, placebo-controlled trial evaluating a drug for severe heart failure (usual care plus active intervention versus usual care plus placebo). A total of 1663 participants enrolled in 16 countries were used in our analysis. We separately analyzed four countries that enrolled more than 100 participants and for which price weights were available (Ns = 130, 372, 382, and 254] plus a miscellaneous category made up of the remaining 12 countries, which in total enrolled 525 participants.

Cost was estimated for hospitalization, active drug therapy, and ambulatory care. Price weights for hospitalization were obtained from four countries that enrolled more than 100 participants, and from one that enrolled fewer. We used the average of price weights collected from four developed countries to value medical service use in seven developed countries for which they were unavailable; we used price weights collected from one developing country to value medical service use in the three developing countries for which they were unavailable.

We report arithmetic mean cost, QALYs, and NMB plus 95% confidence intervals, which we estimated by use of nonparametric bootstrap analyses for both the pooled and country-specific data. We report a pooled result, results for the four countries that enrolled more than 100 participants and for which price weight data were available, and for the miscellaneous category. For NMB, we calculated point estimates and 95% confidence intervals for three values of willingness to pay, 20,000, 50,000, and 80,000. We also report statistical tests of the homogeneity of NMB.

Table 10.2 shows the pooled and country-specific differences in incremental cost and QALYs. For cost, the point estimates for the pooled result and for countries 1 through 4 indicated cost savings, whereas only the point estimate for the miscellaneous category of countries indicated a cost increase. At the same time, none of the six 95% confidence intervals, including that for the pooled result, indicated that we could be confident of savings. For QALYs, every point estimate indicated that the therapy improved the outcome. For the pooled result and two of the countries, the confidence intervals confirmed this finding; for countries C2, C4, and the miscellaneous category, the confidence intervals suggested we could not be confident.

The tests of homogeneity provided no evidence of either qualitative or quantitative interaction. P values ranged from a low of 0.5 for a quantitative interaction for QALYs to a high of 1.0 for a qualitative interaction for QALYs. Thus, we have no evidence that these outcomes differ between the countries.

This finding does not rule out a finding of country-by-treatment heterogeneity for NMB. Table 10.3 shows point estimates and 95% confidence

Table 10.2 Pooled and country-specific estimates of incremental cost and QALYs

	Cost		QALYs	
Country	**Mean**	**95% CI**	**Mean**	**95% CI**
Pooled	−847	−2015 to 316	0.08	0.04 to 0.12
C1	−932	−2647 to 654	0.08	0.01 to 0.16
C2	−802	−4895 to 2872	0.09	−0.02 to 0.22
C3	−452	−3195 to 2606	0.15	0.05 to 0.25
C4	−2457	−6056 to 945	0.06	−0.03 to 0.14
Miscellaneous	283	−1243 to 1869	0.04	−0.01 to 0.10
Qualitative	$p > 0.50$	$p = 1.00$		
Quantitative	$p = 0.65$	$p = 0.50$		

Table 10.3 Pooled and country-specific estimates of net monetary benefits (NMBs) selected ceiling ratios

Country	20,000 Mean	20,000 95% CI	50,000 Mean	50,000 95% CI	80,000 Mean	80,000 95% CI
Pooled	2429	1157 to 3793	4801	2741 to 6953	7174	4171 to 10,389
C1	2509	400 to 4743	4876	768 to 8697	7242	1118 to 13,094
C2	2570	−1959 to 7432	5224	−1521 to 13,073	7877	−1876 to 19,292
C3	3407	−176 to 7029	7838	2037 to 13,836	12,270	3778 to 21,382
C4	3583	26 to 7445	5271	67 to 10,849	6960	−557 to 14,595
Other	556	−1386 to 2461	1814	−1470 to 4983	3072	−1639 to 7888

Tests for interaction

Qualitative	$p= 1.00$		$p= 1.00$		$p = 1.00$	
Quantitative	$p = 0.51$		$p = 0.40$		$p = 0.43$	

intervals for the pooled and country-specific estimates of NMB. All point estimates for all three values of willingness to pay are positive. Depending upon the willingness to pay, the confidence intervals for the pooled result and for two or three of the five countries confirmed this finding. For the remaining one or two countries, the confidence intervals indicated we could not be confident of savings.

However, as with cost and QALYs, the heterogeneity tests provided no evidence of either qualitative or quantitative interaction. Thus, if we believe the tests are sufficiently powered, we cannot reject that the pooled result, suggesting significant positive NMB, applies to all of the countries that participated in the trial.

How should we interpret these findings? In the example, we found little evidence of between-country differences in the incremental cost, QALYs, and NMB associated with therapy for severe heart failure. In this case, we may want to use the more precise trial-wide estimate for each of the countries in the trial. This pooled point estimate suggests that usual care plus active therapy was cost effective compared with usual care alone because the lower limit of the 95% confidence interval for NMB was 1157 when calculated by use of a willingness to pay of 20,000.

Could there be a difference in the country-specific results that we did not detect? We cannot rule out such a possibility, given that the power of the test for homogeneity is low. However, at worst the evidence is that we cannot distinguish the value for the cost of the two therapies.

Addressing Power

As we have noted throughout this discussion, homogeneity tests are well known for being low powered. One approach to overcoming this problem is to use larger α levels (e.g., 0.1 or 0.2) and look for larger differences between groups. A second is to pool countries across relevant attributes. For example, one might pool countries with similar practice characteristics (e.g., types of centers and providers or characteristics of reimbursement systems). Ex post, one might pool countries with most similar results, to determine whether there might be sets of countries in which there are systematic differences for the economic results. The principle underlying these latter hypothesis generating tests is that given the tests tend toward a finding of homogeneity, we should try to identify any evidence of heterogeneity that may exist.

10.3.3. Multilevel models with random effects empirical Bayesian shrinkage estimators

An alternative to homogeneity tests is to use multilevel random effects models. Multilevel models account for the hierarchical structure of data (i.e., the fact that patients are treated by physicians in centers which means that these data may violate the assumption that the random errors are independently distributed). These models have been widely used in fields such as education and health services research [21,22], and have been used more recently to analyze cost data from multinational randomized trials [13,14], to estimate incremental net benefits across centers [12], and to compare medical service use and cost across health care providers [23–25]. These models specifically account for the fact that when we subdivide a larger group into subgroups, we expect that the point estimates will vary even when all of the subgroups have been drawn from the same underlying population (i.e., homogeneity).

As Manca *et al.* [12] have demonstrated, multilevel random effects models provide more precise estimates of country-specific results than those resulting from analysis of each country's data separately and provide unbiased standard errors. These models can also be used to generate country-specific cost-effectiveness estimates by use of empirical Bayesian shrinkage estimation, a feature available in multilevel models.

The empirical Bayesian shrinkage estimator is a weighted sum of the estimates provided by the pooled random effects estimate (i.e., that lump the estimates across country) and the country-specific observed difference (i.e., that splits the estimates by country) [14]. It has been given the name "shrinkage estimator" because the resulting weighted averages are closer to the pooled estimate than are the observed country-specific differences (i.e., they are shrunk towards the pooled result). The shrinkage estimator is made up of the between-country variability and the N-weighted within-country variability. The amount of information "borrowed" (i.e., "shrinkage") from the pooled estimate depends on the relative magnitudes of the two sources of variance and the sample size in the country. The smaller the between-country variance relative to the within-country variance or the smaller the N, the more the estimates of the country-specific difference are shrunken towards the pooled random effects estimate across all countries [13].

Use of this approach improves statistical efficiency by borrowing information from all countries in the estimation of country-specific differences [14]. Pinto *et al.* [13] have proposed the use of shrinkage estimation for both cost and effectiveness to provide a more efficient country-specific cost-effectiveness analysis than is provided by the use of country-specific data alone. In their article, the authors proposed a series of univariate and multivariable shrinkage estimators and evaluated their performance by use of simulation. They demonstrated that in the presence of between-country heterogeneity, the random effects pooled estimator is a poor estimator of country-specific effects. They also showed that the shrinkage estimators achieved a substantial reduction [20–59%] in average standard error compared to the error without shrinkage. For example, they found that shrinkage estimators reduced the standard error for the Canadian estimate by 33% compared with the standard error that resulted from the Canadian data alone. The authors calculated that in order to achieve the same level of precision by use of the latter data alone would have required more than twice the sample size in Canada.

The advantages of such multilevel models are their correct handling of the clustered data and their ability to use information from all countries to produce shrunken country-specific estimates. One of the assumptions that underlie the validity of these latter estimates, however, is that the quantities being estimated in different countries are "exchangeable." By exchangeable we mean that prior to the trial, we have no a priori information suggesting that particular countries are likely to have better or worse cost-effectiveness than others [12,14,26]. The validity of this assumption may be questioned, particularly given that it seems to prejudge the answer to questions about transferability.

A related set of assumptions of multilevel models is that the true country-specific means are drawn from a normal distribution and that the mean and variance of this distribution are common to all countries [13]. Willan *et al.* [14] have noted that these may be strong assumptions whose validity cannot rely on the central limit theorem. For example, Pinto *et al.* [13] have suggested that in some circumstances, structural differences between countries may imply that the assumption of a common mean is not realistic, and it will be appropriate to differentiate between, for example, the means for developing and developed countries. In such a case, an indicator variable representing type of country can be added to the model, and the empirical Bayesian estimates can be shrunken towards two separate pooled means, one for developing countries and one for developed [13].

Willan *et al.* [14] and Pinto *et al.* [13] have argued that the normality assumption itself may not be as problematic. They point out that we make the normality assumption for many of the methods we use in the estimation of cost-effectiveness and its sampling uncertainty, and that – in light of the central limit theorem – the results are robust even when the patient-level observations are quite skewed.

Pietz [27], on the other hand, has indicated that the best linear unbiased predictions (BLUPs) derived from multilevel random effects models are less robust to departures from normality than are the best linear unbiased estimates (BLUEs) yielded by fixed effects models that have the Gauss–Markov theorem as their basis. Nixon and Thompson [28] and Thompson *et al.* [26] have proposed that analysts explicitly address the skewness of cost or cost-effectiveness data in hierarchical or multilevel models. Thompson, *et al.* [26] used generalized linear multilevel models to estimate the effects of patient and national characteristics on costs. They found that the use of methods such as a generalized linear multilevel model with a gamma distribution and log link accounted not only for the clustering in the data, but also for differences in the skewness and variance of the data across countries. Their GLM model fit the data better than other multilevel models that assumed normal distributions or estimated additive effects. Nixon and Thompson [28] presented a similar generalized linear model approach for the bivariate analysis of cost-effectiveness in the context of multicenter-randomized trials.

Finally, Willan *et al.* [14] have noted that while Bayesian shrinkage estimates can be used to provide center-specific estimates in a multicenter trial within a country or region, the analysis of such multicenter trials is probably best based on the overall random effects estimate. They base this argument on the observation that policy decisions on adoption of treatments are more often made at the regional or national level rather than at the center level.

10.4. **Potential problems common to all three methods**

While these three methods differ in their approach to answering questions of transferability, there are at least five potential problems that are common to all of them.

10.4.1. **Protocol effects and transferability**

All three analytic approaches evaluate the similarities and differences between country-specific results as if they arose naturally and independently from the trial. However, as we discussed in Chapter 2, trial protocols often try to standardize the care of participants who participate in the trial. To the extent that these protocols are successful, any findings of homogeneity, or dramatic shrinkage towards the pooled result, may simply be an artifact of this standardization. We should be most confident that the protocol is not artificially driving a finding of transferability when we observe between-country variability in medical service use in the placebo group (implying a protocol that is not strongly homogenizing care), yet we are able to observe common cost-effectiveness across the countries. We should be least confident when there is little or no between-country variability in medical service use in the placebo group – which raises the question of whether the protocol has strongly homogenized care in the trial – and we observe similar cost-effectiveness in each country. For example, Cook *et al.* [11] reported that hospitalization rates differed between the five countries they evaluated, but they were unable to detect any heterogeneity in the treatment's effect on hospitalization rates.

10.4.2. **Influential observations**

As we noted in Chapter 5, evaluation of the pooled average effect of therapy on cost is complicated by the existence of a small number of observations with extreme values for cost (i.e., their existence is one of the reasons why some investigators abandon the arithmetic mean, and instead evaluate medians or transformed cost). If these observations pose problems when we are evaluating the pooled treatment effect, consider the problems they pose for the analysis of country-specific treatment effect. These few observations will often be spread, possibly one each, across several countries. Their existence will make it difficult for us to determine whether observed homogeneity or country-specific differences are due to these individual observations or whether they are due to underlying differences between the countries. See Langford and Lewis [29] for an extended discussion on the diagnosis and handling of outliers in multilevel models.

10.4.3. Transferability and censored data

As we indicated in Chapter 6, the principle that underlies most methods for addressing censored data is to "borrow" data – either by inverse probability weighting or multiple imputation – from participants who are "like" participants whose data are censored. The question that underlies the issue of transferability, on the other hand, is whether the data from participants from one country are representative of data from participants from another country. Thus, if we "borrow" data from different countries to address censoring, it is an open question whether we will undermine our ability to detect country-specific differences.

10.4.4. Sample size

Many multinational trials now enroll participants in 40 or 50 countries, and for many of these countries only 10 or 15 participants are enrolled. Such a design poses problems for all three methods, although not necessarily equally (i.e., shrinkage estimates may not be as affected by small sample sizes per country, although small sample sizes predisposes one towards large amounts of shrinkage to the mean). For example, when we test homogeneity, small samples in each country will generally yield large country-specific confidence intervals for NMB. Large intervals make rejection of homogeneity of the treatment effect difficult.

One means of overcoming this problem is to modify the trial design so that more participants are enrolled in fewer countries. If it is infeasible to change the trial design, as we discussed earlier, we may want to change the level of analysis for the homogeneity test. For example, we may want to aggregate across "similar" countries, where similarity might be defined by level of economic development, practice pattern, or characteristics of the health care reimbursement system. We would then evaluate the homogeneity of the economic impact for these larger groups of participants rather than evaluating the impact between countries.

10.4.5. Countries that did not participate in the trial

Finally, none of the three methods directly provide information for countries that did not participate in the trial. There has been little published methodologic work for addressing this problem, and without knowing the specifics of any particular country, it is hard to generalize. Decision analysis is one option for attempting to address this issue. Another approach may be to identify countries that participated in the trial that are similar to those that did not, and use the information from the one to inform decisions for the other.

10.5. **Summary**

Issues of transferability are of growing importance as decision makers in more countries seek information about the likely economic impact of the adoption of new therapies in their countries. Historically, we have tended to do a poor job of estimation of transferability: although we seem to focus most on adjusting price weights, they likely are not the primary source of variability when countries have similar economic conditions.

Three recently proposed analytic techniques provide improved methods for addressing issues of transferability: fixed effects models, tests of homogeneity, and multilevel random effects models. Each method uses data from the trial to address these issues. Our early understanding is that the methods trade-off problems of power for problems of exchangeability.

In many trials, small sample sizes may limit our ability to detect country-specific effects, no matter which method we pursue in the evaluation of transferability. In these cases, we may be better served to look at major contrasts that provide some, but not necessarily all, of the information sought by decision makers. Does the therapy compliment other supportive care (i.e., is it more cost-effective when this care is present) or does it substitute for other supportive care (i.e., is it more cost-effective in the absence of this care)? If the trial is conducted in countries with a mix of levels of development, is the therapy more or less cost-effective in developed countries than it is in developing countries? Simply knowing these relationships should improve our understanding of the transferability of the economic results from multinational trials.

References

1. O'Brien BS. A tale of two (or more) cities: geographic transferability of pharmacoeconomic data. *Am J Manage Care* 1997; 3: S33–40.
2. Willke RJ, Glick HA, Polsky D, Schulman K. Estimating country-specific cost-effectiveness from multinational clinical trials. *Health Econ.* 1998; 7: 481–93.
3. Glick HA, Polsky D, Willke RJ, Alves WM, Kassell N, Schulman K. Comparison of the use of medical resources and outcomes in the treatment of aneurysmal subarachnoid hemorrhage between Canada and the United States. *Stroke* 1998; 29: 351–8.
4. Commonwealth of Australia. Guidelines for the Pharmaceutical Industry on Preparation of Submissions to the Pharmaceutical Benefits Advisory Committee. Canberra: Department of Health and Community Services, 1995.
5. Canadian Coordinating Office for Health Technology Assessment. Guidelines for Economic Evaluation of Pharmaceuticals: Canada, 2nd ed. Ottawa: Canadian Coordinating Office for Health Technology Assessment (CCOHTA), 1997.
6. National Institute for Clinical Guidance. Guidance for Manufacturers and Sponsors. Technology Appraisals Process Series No. 5. London: National Institute for Clinical Excellence, 2001.

7. Reed SD, Anstrom KJ, Bakhai A, Briggs AH, Califf RM, Cohen DJ, Drummond MF, Glick HA, Gnanasakthy A, Hlatky MA, O'Brien BJ, Torti FM, Tsiatis AA, Willan AR, Mark DB, Schulman KA. Conducting economic evaluations alongside multinational clinical trials: toward a research consensus. *Am Heart J*. 2005; 149: 434–43.

8. Barbieri M, Drummond M, Willke R, Chancellor, J, Jolain B, Towse A. Variability of cost-effectiveness estimates for pharmaceuticals in Western Europe: lessons for inferring generalizability. *Value Health* 2005; 8: 10–23.

9. Office of Health Economics. OHE-Health Economic Evaluation Database. London: OHE, 2002.

10. NHS Centre for Reviews and Dissemination. NHS Economic Evaluation Database. York: NHS CRD, 2002.

11. Cook JR, Drummond MR, Glick H, Heyse JF. Assessing the appropriateness of combining economic data from multinational clinical trials. *Stat Med*. 2003; 22: 1955–76.

12. Manca A, Rice N, Sculpher MJ, Briggs AH. Assessing generalisability by location in trial-based cost-effectiveness analysis: the use of multilevel models. *Health Econ*. 2005; 14: 471–85.

13. Pinto EM, Willan AR, O'Brien BJ. Cost-effectiveness analysis for multinational clinical trials. *Stat Med*. 2005; 24: 1965–82.

14. Willan AR, Pinto EM, O'Brien BJ, Kaul P, Goeree R, Lynd L, Armstrong PW. Country specific cost comparisons from multinational clinical trials using empirical Bayesian shrinkage estimation: the Canadian ASSENT-3 economic analysis. *Health Econ*. 2005; 14: 327–38.

15. Drummond MF, Bloom BS, Carrin G, Hillman AL, Hutchings HC, Knill-Jones RP, de Pouvourville G, Torfs K. Issues in the cross-national assessment of health technology. *Int J Tech Assess Health Care* 1992; 8: 671–82.

16. Menzin J, Oster G, Davies L, Drummond M, Greiner W, Merot J-L, Rossi F, Graf v.d. Schulenberg J, Souetre E. A multinational economic evaluation of rhDNase in the treatment of cystic fibrosis. *Intl J Tech Assess Health Care* 1996; 12: 52–61.

17. Jonsson B, Weinstein WC. Economic evaluation alongside multinational clinical trials: study considerations for GUSTO IIb. *Intl J Tech Assess Health Care* 1997; 13: 49–58.

18. Gail M, Simon R. Testing for qualitative interactions between treatment effects and patient subsets. *Biometrics* 1985; 41: 361–72.

19. Peto R. Statistical aspects of cancer trials. In Treatment of Cancer, edited by K.E. Halnan.London: Chapman and Hall, 1982, pp. 867–71.

20. Pan G, Wolfe DA. Test for qualitative interaction of clinical significance. *Stat Med*. 1997; 16: 1645–52.

21. Goldstein H. Multilevel Statistical Models. London: Edward Arnold, 1995

22. Leyland AH, Goldstein H (editors). Multi-level Modelling of Health Statistics. Chichester: Wiley, 2001.

23. Grieve R, Nixon R, Thompson SG, Normand C. Using multilevel models for assessing the variability of multinational resource use and cost data. *Health Econ*. 2005; 14: 185–96.

24. Burgess JE, Cristiansen CL, Michalak SE, Morris CN. Medical profiling: improving standards and risk adjustments using hierarchical models. *J Health Econ*. 2000; 19: 291–309.

25. Carey K. A multi-level modelling approach to analysis of patient costs under managed care. *Health Econ.* 2000; 9: 435–46.

26. Thompson SG, Nixon RM, Grieve R. Addressing the issues that arise in analysing multicentre cost data, with application to a multinational study. *J Health Econ.* 2006; 25:1015–28.

27. Pietz K. An introduction to hierarchical models. February, 2003. www.hsrd.houston.med.va. gov/Linear%20Models.ppt.

28. Nixon RM, Thompson SG. Incorporating covariate adjustment, subgroup analysis and between-centre differences into cost-effectiveness evaluations. *Health Econ.* 2005; 14: 1217–29.

29. Langford IH, Lewis T. Outliers in multilevel data. *J R Stat Soc A.* 1998; 161: 121–60.

Chapter 11

Relevance of trial-based economic analyses

Our goal has been to provide you with an in-depth understanding of economic assessment conducted by use of patient-level data collected as part of randomized controlled trials. To this end, we have discussed issues relevant to the design and conduct of such assessments (Chapter 2), the identification of appropriate sets of price weights (Chapter 3), the measurement of quality-adjusted life years (Chapter 4), the analysis of cost in the absence (Chapter 5) and presence (Chapter 6) of censored data, the comparison of cost and effect (Chapter 7), and the assessment of sampling uncertainty (Chapters 8 and 9) and transferability (Chapter 10) of this comparison.

Use of the techniques we have described in combination with other good practice guidelines for the conduct of randomized trials will produce internally valid estimates of the cost-effectiveness of the therapies evaluated in the trial which can be reported in the same manner as the estimates of clinical efficacy or effectiveness that are derived from the trial. As with the reporting of clinical efficacy, any comparison of cost-effectiveness should include estimates of sampling uncertainty as well as the equivalent of tests of homogeneity of the economic outcome. As trialists, producing these estimates may be the principal goal of our economic evaluation, in the same way that a clinical scientist's goal may be to evaluate the clinical outcomes resulting from a therapy.

As we indicated in Chapter 1, however, one of the reasons we undertake economic evaluation is to inform the policy debate about whether a clinically safe and effective therapy provides sufficient value for its cost to be adopted for use. Until now, we have said nothing about the relevance of the cost-effectiveness results from trials to this policy debate. In what follows, we address this question of relevance by posing a series of questions and then answering them.

1. *What are the attributes of trials that make them more relevant to the policy debate?*

    (A) *Adopt a cost-effective comparator* – One concern that is often raised about trial-based analyses is that trials rarely compare the study therapy to all potential alternative therapy options. On this line of reasoning, a trial may demonstrate cost-effectiveness against the comparator used in the trial, but that does not mean it has demonstrated cost-effectiveness against other potential comparators.

One means of addressing this problem is to adopt a comparator in the trial that is a well-accepted therapeutic choice for which there is good evidence of its cost-effectiveness compared to other potential alternatives. We recommend adoption of such a comparator because if the comparator is cost-effective compared to the alternatives, and if we can demonstrate that the new therapy is cost-effective compared to the comparator, it follows that the new therapy is cost-effective compared to the alternatives. A proof of this claim can be derived from the mathematics that underlies the algorithm for identifying the therapy with an acceptable ratio when more than two therapies are compared (see Table 7.2, Chapter 7).

(B) *Adopt a final outcome such as QALYs* – As we indicated in Chapter 2, use of intermediate outcomes such as illness days avoided or abstinence days for which standards of willingness to pay are not routinely available may make the results of trials less relevant to the policy debate. This is particularly true if the trial failed to use QALYs because its timeframe was too short to see an improvement in this outcome.

(C) *Enroll a representative sample of the patient population who will use the therapy* – Trials often use highly specialized patient populations, e.g., those at very high risk, who have a large enough event rate that the trial can be conducted in a timely fashion. At the same time, sponsors often would like to use the results from trials that enroll these specialized patient populations to justify use of the therapy in more general, lower risk populations.

As we pointed out in Chapter 10, the problem with generalizing cost-effectiveness observed in high-risk populations to low-risk populations is that cost-effectiveness is based on absolute, not relative effects of therapy. Thus, if the underlying event rate in the more general population is lower than the event rate observed in the high-risk population that was enrolled in the trial, we would expect that the cost-effectiveness of the new therapy, when used in the broader population, would be less favorable than it was in the trial. One way to overcome this problem is to perform trials in populations like those that will use the therapy in usual care. A more speculative approach might be to perform a weighted analysis of the trial data, the weights of which are used to rebalance the risk groups observed in the trial so that they are more reflective of the risks in the general patient population. In essence, we up-weight lower risk participants and down-weight higher risk participants.

(D) *Adopt a sufficiently long period of follow-up* – Mortality trials, in which a substantial fraction of participants die, are the trials most likely to have a direct effect on the policy debate. If 40–50% of participants die, if the new therapy can be shown to be cost-effective, and if – as was the case in Table 2.1 in Chapter 2 – the trajectory of cost-effectiveness is improving throughout the trial, it is unlikely that nontrial-based analyses, such as decision models, will be able to demonstrate lack of cost-effectiveness.

This observation does not mean that mortality trials are the only ones in which the cost-effectiveness outcome may be relevant to the policy debate. For example, trials of a quality of life-enhancing therapy that demonstrate a sustained annual benefit of, for example, 0.05 QALYs and an annual incremental cost of 500 (10,000 per QALY) may also be convincing by themselves.

One of the presumptions that appears to underlie the issue of the (in)adequacy of the time horizons in trials is that there necessarily is a treatment-by-time interaction for cost-effectiveness. In other words, there is a presumption that cost-effectiveness ratios are either always improving or worsening with longer periods of follow-up. The implication of this presumption is that lifetime projections are necessary for understanding the impact of medical therapies that (1) are used for chronic conditions or (2) are for short-term conditions but affect survival.

We are not confident that this presumption is correct. As we indicated in Chapter 2, if follow-up in the trial is sufficiently long, by the end of the trial the observed cost-effectiveness ratio may already be asymptotically approaching the long-term cost-effectiveness ratio. Furthermore, even if the period of follow-up within the trial is not sufficiently long, asymptotic progress may occur after only 5 or 10 years of projection of the results. Thus, given that the "model" uncertainty that surrounds 30- and 40-year projections is substantially greater than that which surrounds 5- and 10-year projections, the possibility of use of shorter modeling periods allows greater confidence in our results.

(E) *Enroll a sufficient number of participants to adequately power the trial* – If the therapy increases both cost and effect, a sufficient number of patients should be enrolled so that the resulting confidence intervals for the cost-effectiveness ratio or for NMB allow decision makers to be confident about the value claim (see formulas for sample size and power in Chapter 9). If, on the other hand, the therapy is cost neutral but more effective or is effect neutral but less costly, do not conflate "absence of evidence" with "evidence of absence" (see discussion in Chapter 9).

(F) *Collect data on a sufficiently broad set of medical services* – To be confident that the cost difference observed in the trial will represent the actual cost difference experienced by participants, we should collect data on a sufficiently broad set of medical services, in a broad range of delivery settings, among all or – if the cost outcome is more than adequately powered – a random sample of trial participants. If we instead focus on a very limited set of services, it will remain an open question whether differences in the services we did not observe could overwhelm the differences we did observe.

(G) *Do not overly prescribe medical care* – As we discussed in Chapter 2, protocol-mandated testing can lead to the detection, and thus treatment, of a greater number of outcomes than would be detected in usual care and can alter the severity of the outcomes at the time of their detection. Protocol-mandated intensive treatment of outcomes will tend to improve the cost-effectiveness of the therapy with the greater number of these outcomes if the mandated treatment is itself cost-effective; it will diminish the cost-effectiveness of this therapy if the mandated treatment is itself not cost-effective. In an effort to avoid the introduction of these biases, trials should be as naturalistic as the regulatory process allows.

(H) *Collect data to assess/improve transferability* – As we discussed in Chapter 10, a major hurdle for the interpretation of the results of trial-based evaluations arises when little if any of these data are collected in the jurisdiction in which the adoption decision is being considered. As we also discussed in that chapter, ideally we would use data from the trial to evaluate country-specific cost-effectiveness, but inadequate sample size and large variability can make estimation of valid and precise estimates for participating countries difficult. It is even more difficult to provide country-specific estimates for countries that did not participate in the trial. As one means of overcoming this hurdle, we have recommended use of data from the trial to assess two major contrasts: (1) Does the therapy compliment or substitute for other supportive care, i.e., is it more or less cost-effective when this care is present? (2) Is the therapy more or less cost-effective in developed countries than it is in developing countries? Answering these

questions may provide decision makers with some of the information they need to judge the cost-effectiveness in their country.

(I) *Observe a sufficiently large or small treatment benefit* – Of course the magnitude of the outcome is not under our control, but all else equal, when the treatment benefits are large, it is easier to demonstrate cost-effectiveness. When the treatment benefits are small, it is easier to observe lack of cost-effectiveness. Thus, the magnitude of the observed benefit plays a role in whether trial-based data are likely to be relevant to the policy debate.

Reading this list, you may come to the conclusion that only a large, multi-year, well-performed, and well-analyzed trial can be relevant to the policy debate. This is not the case, in part because evidence from trials is not all or none, but instead is more or less. Each of these attributes is represented by a continuum ranging from their being poorly met to their being well met. The evidence from trials is stronger when they better meet more of these attributes rather than fewer. Or to put it more directly, many trials have had sufficient evidence to make important contributions to adoption decisions without being conducted with thousands of participants and a follow-up of 10 years.

2. *What are the attributes of trials that make them less relevant to the policy debate?*

The converse of all these nine attributes all decreases the relevance of the evidence from trials to the policy debate. Other features that undermine their relevance include the use of inappropriate statistical tests and the reporting of inappropriate moments of the distribution, failure to adequately address problems arising from missing data, and lack of an intention-to-treat analysis. For example, in a recent review of eight reports on cost-effectiveness from six trials of second-generation antipsychotics, Polsky *et al.*[1] concluded that the investigators did not adequately address a number of these 12 issues, which led their cost-effectiveness claims to be unconvincing.

3. *Is it illegitimate to report the cost-effectiveness ratio observed in a trial without performing a broader decision analysis or systematic review of the data?*

This question may be unexpected, but some have argued that the principal role of trials is to measure economic (and clinical?) parameters that can be used in systematic reviews and decision analysis [2]. On this interpretation, one might ask whether it is legitimate to report the cost-effectiveness ratio observed in a trial.

We do not see economic data collected within a trial as being different in kind from clinical data. Investigators routinely report clinical results of trials without being required to perform a systematic review that explains how the current trial result changes the state of our knowledge. In the same way that the clinical result describes what was observed in the trial, the cost-effectiveness ratio and its confidence interval also describes what was observed in the trial. It is not clear why the reporting principles that are appropriate for clinical results would not also be appropriate for economic results. Thus, we consider it appropriate to report the cost-effectiveness ratio observed in a trial without simultaneously reporting a broader decision analysis or systematic review.

Furthermore, to suppose that every group of investigators who perform a clinical trial should develop a decision model or systematic review is an inefficient use of research funding. It would be better for investigators who specialize in decision analysis or systematic reviews to incorporate the results of the trial into their models and reviews than it would be to require that every clinical trial report such a synthesis. At the same time, as the ISPOR RCT-CEA Task Force [3] has recommended, if we want the economic data to be available for synthesis, "authors should report means and standard errors for the incremental costs and outcomes and their correlation" (p. 528).

4. *Should evidence from a single trial-based economic evaluation stand alone as evidence of the value for the cost for the adoption decision?*

Regulatory agencies such as the U.S. Food and Drug administration usually require evidence from two well-designed trials before they recognize a clinical claim about a new therapy. To continue the analogy with clinical evidence, it is again not clear why we would want to relax this standard.

5. *Could evidence from two well-designed trials be sufficient for the adoption decision?*

Under certain circumstances, yes, evidence from two well-designed trials could be sufficient for the adoption decision. For example, the clinical evidence from within the trials might be so compelling and the evidence of value might be so strong that little, if any, additional evidence would be needed. For example, if each of the two 4-year follow-up trials found that therapy yielded approximately 0.25 QALYs (95% CI, 0.1–0.4) compared to a well-recognized, cost-effective comparator and that it reduced hospitalization sufficiently to offset its cost, it is unlikely that any additional information could modify the adoption decision.

To put this answer more technically, the cost-effectiveness evidence from the trials may be so strong that a value of information analysis [4] would indicate that no further evidence gathering, decision analysis, or synthesis is required for the adoption decision.

6. *What are the roles of trial-based and model-based evidence?*

The fact that trial-based evidence could be sufficient for the adoption decision does not mean that it, routinely, will be sufficient. When it is not, in some cases a combination of trial- and model-based evidence may be sufficient. In others, as Sculpher *et al.* [2] have suggested, the results of the trial might serve simply as inputs to decision analysis.

Our principal concern is with the presumption that trial-based evaluation is irrelevant to the policy decision. It is easy to propose what appears to be very reasonable, but are in fact very stringent, requirements for decision making [2], particularly when there is no balancing of the strengths and weaknesses of different sources of evidence. Real-world decision making is based on bounded rationality and satisficing [5,6], and not hyperrationality. Thus, the requirements of decision making should not be whether we have considered all of everything or whether the omission of some piece of evidence might lead to "a partial analysis with potentially misleading results" [2, p. 679], but instead should be whether we have considered enough of everything. That is why we have argued that there are limited instances in which the evidence from trials can be strong enough that decisions can be made based on them alone.

We believe that both trial-based data and decision models have strengths and weaknesses, and that rather than debating about "evidence" versus "a source of parameter estimates," we should realistically weigh these strengths and weaknesses. Yes, trials do not answer all of our questions, and we should always be aware of their limitations in terms of patient populations, comparators, settings, and the like. Yes, decision models may be more conjecture than they are evidence, and we should always be aware that the simple fact that they produce projections does not make them good or accurate ones. One reason economists believe that more information is better than less is because they assume that its disposal is costless. Finally, yes, notions of bounded rationality and satisficing support our use of both sources of evidence for decision making even though we do not "know" that either provides an accurate answer to our questions.

Thus, in closing, we repeat our recommendation that economic data from within a trial should be analyzed and reported in a manner similar to analysis and reporting of clinical data. We should also report the data in ways that it will be usable for data synthesis. As with most human endeavors, there are many ways of knowing.

References

1. Polsky D, Doshi JA, Bauer MS, Glick HA. Clinical Trial-Based Cost-Effectiveness Analyses of Antipsychotics. *Am J Psychiatry*. In press.
2. Sculpher MJ, Claxton K, Drummond M, McCabe C. Whither trial-based economic evaluation for health care decision making? *Health Econ*. 2006; 15: 677–87.
3. Ramsey S, Willke R, Briggs A, Brown R, Buxton M, Chawla A, Cook J, Glick H, Liljas B, Petitti D, Reed S. Best Practices for economic analysis alongside clinical trials: an ISPOR RCT-CEA Task Force report. *Value Health*. 2005; 8: 521–33.

4. Claxton K, Ginnelly L, Sculpher M, Philips Z, Palmer S, A pilot study on the use of decision theory and value of information analysis as part of the National Health Service Health Technology Assessment Programme. *Health Technol Assess.* 2004; 8: 1–132.
5. Simon HA. A behavioral model of rational choice. *Quarterly Econ.* 1955; 69: 99–118.
6. Kahnman D. Maps of bounded rationality: psychology for behavioral economics. *Am Econ Rev.* 2003; 93: 1449–75.

Index